Calming Guillain-Barré

Calming Guillain-Barré

Nancy Mount

To order additional copies of this book, contact:
Xlibris Corporation
1-888-795-4274
www.Xlibris.com
Orders@Xlibris.com
92034

CONTENTS

Part IV

You as Healer: Putting Out the Fire

INTRODUCTION

THIS BOOK IS intended for Guillain-Barré syndrome (GBS) patients and recoverers, their family members, friends, and other support people who want to know all they can about GBS. It is written for the purpose of summarizing as much information as possible about GBS basics and ways to promote recovery. In an effort to present the most up-to-date, hundreds of recent medical research reports have been screened to filter out the most relevant and helpful breaking news about GBS in a very readable style for the average person. What makes this GBS book different from others is that it is an evidence-based self-help book for GBS recoverers.

GBS victims, their loved ones, and others connected to their lives hunger for information about this condition, which comes on so suddenly, turning ordinary lives upside down. Seeking knowledge is a natural instinct because it gives us power over the unknown. Knowledge about what may be expected and what can be done better helps to make informed decisions and to remove the fear of the unknown. Yet in the prognosis of GBS, much remains unknown. One of the most formidable pieces of information given to the GBS patient is that there is no known cure—that is, there is no pill or treatment that will take the affliction away. Also, there are the unknowns of how extensive and how severe the symptoms will progress. Possibly, the most worrisome unknown is the recovery phase. Although most GBS victims do recover, the length of time and the degree of recovery cannot be predicted with any degree of certainty.

This book can make a huge difference in the approach to GBS recovery as viewed through the eyes of the patient. Although conventional care involves follow-up checkups and physical therapy, recovery is a passive time of waiting to heal. In contrast, based on scientific evidence, this book presents safe and practical ways for the patient to take an active role in recovery. Supporting documentation is given here for three natural ways to lessen inflammation and to potentially improve the outcome of GBS.

By implementing a dietary regimen that is consistently full of antioxidants and empty of the types of foods that promote inflammation, by taking antioxidant supplements, and by practicing a daily routine of Breath Work, the GBS recoverer may start to feel the benefits within a short period of time. As stated throughout this book, it is important to always seek the approval of the attending physician before implementing any new routine to ensure that dietary changes, supplements, and Breath Work practice do not interfere with conventional medical care.

As a chemist and as a natural health professional, I have been studying antioxidants and their role in counteracting inflammation for some time. Inflammation left unchecked causes premature aging, pain, and chronic diseases and conditions, all costing us great amounts of money and lost quality of life. In my lifetime, I have personally known brave victims battling neuropathies, such as multiple sclerosis, transverse myelitis, amylotrophic lateral sclerosis, and myasthenia gravis. When a friend of the family, a young father who was previously in excellent health, was suddenly paralyzed by what was eventually diagnosed as GBS, I was moved to find out all I could about it and to write a book that could help those suffering with GBS. My research led me to discover that inflammation is the common link in those neuropathies and that a flood of free radicals are involved in initiating the cascade of chemicals in the body that causes the destruction of healthy nerves. It was logical, then, to look for relevant research in the potential therapeutic use of antioxidants in GBS because antioxidants quench free radicals by absorbing the unpaired electron, which makes them so reactive.

The research process of this book was extremely interesting and rewarding. I even learned that the acute symmetrical progression of numbness, joint swelling, pain, and partial paralysis in addition to headache, fever, and insomnia, which I had experienced years ago, were probably symptoms of a bout of GBS, secondary to exposure to a virus. At that time, and after several office calls, my doctor was baffled, so he sent me to a rheumatologist, who ran a panel of blood tests. Results showed that I had elevated levels of parvovirus antibodies. But it was now nearly two months later, and by the time the blood tests came back, my symptoms were subsiding. Interestingly, my research for this book revealed several case reports that parvovirus can be a GBS trigger although I was never diagnosed with GBS. What I remembered most about this time was my frustration in not knowing what was going on while I progressively got worse. My reaction was to read everything I could find that might explain my seemingly hopeless condition. By reading *Calming Guillain-Barre'*, the GBS patient will not only be better able to communicate and make informed decisions along with conventional medical care specialists; he or she can also take action to promote healing with "Superfoods," antioxidant supplements, and Breath Work. Where there is knowledge, there is hope.

PART I

Guillain-Barré Syndrome Basics

CHAPTER 1

What is Guillain-Barré Syndrome?

An Autoimmune Attack on the Peripheral Nervous System

SCIENTISTS NOW KNOW that Guillain-Barré syndrome (GBS) is a disorder of the immune system. It is most often associated with a recent infection or exposure to a virus, bacteria, or other antigen. In GBS, the result is acute inflammation of the peripheral nerves leading to their degeneration, a condition referred to as acute peripheral neuropathy. When working properly, the immune system maintains an inflammatory response to keep foreign invaders from becoming established, even keeping newly forming cancer cells in check. However, during the autoimmune response, white blood cells that initiate inflammation are "tricked" into thinking that normal body cells are foreign because they chemically resemble what the body has come to recognize as the surface molecules of the invading virus or bacteria. In an autoimmune response, inflammation initiates the destruction of healthy, normal body cells and tissues.

The nervous system is made up of two distinct parts: the central nervous system and the peripheral nervous system. The central nervous system is composed of the brain and the spinal cord. Peripheral nerves extend from the central nervous system to the head, the arms, the legs, and the body. GBS is generally categorized as a type of peripheral neuropathy with a collection of distinguishing symptoms. Due to the sudden onset of symptoms, which progress over a period of several days to a few weeks, it is called an acute peripheral neuropathy. Although GBS is considered to be rare, affecting on the average only two out of one hundred thousand people worldwide, it is the most common reason for acute paralysis in this country.

GBS Symptoms Are Acute

Shortly after symptoms of the triggering infection have disappeared or after exposure to an antigen, scientific studies indicate that in GBS the immune system begins to attack healthy fibers of the peripheral nervous system. One of the distinguishing characteristics of GBS is that it typically comes on suddenly—that is, it has *acute* onset. Usually within a period of a few days to several weeks, a gradual symmetrical weakness is experienced in the hands, the feet, or the head, often spreading to other parts of the body in a descending or ascending progression. It is common to have unusual sensations prior to the recognized weakness. These sensations are medically referred to as paresthesias, and they include feelings such as tingling, numbness, prickling, cramping, and pain. If muscles to the diaphragm become involved, this is of primary medical concern since breathing assistance may be required, and the patient must be hospitalized. In some types of GBS, nerves to the head and neck area may be affected, which can result in symptoms such as blurred vision, a loss of the sense of smell, slurred speech, an inability to move facial muscles, and difficulty in swallowing.

Basic GBS Classifications

If you imagine a string of oblong beads as a mental picture of a peripheral nerve fiber, the "string" could represent the nerve axon, and the "beads" would be the segments of the myelin sheath. Axons can also be thought of as electrical wires because they conduct electrical signals throughout the nervous system, and they are most vulnerable at the junctions between the bead-like segments of myelin. The myelin sheath segments serve to insulate the axon to prevent electricity from leaking out into surrounding fluids, causing a short circuit. When the myelin is destroyed, the resulting degeneration is called demyelination.

GBS is classified into two main types: *Axonal* GBS is reported to be more common in developing countries where it is mostly associated with contaminated drinking water. The other main type, *demyelinating* GBS—referred to as acute inflammatory demyelinating neuropathy, or AIDP—is the most prevalent type of GBS worldwide, and it is the most common type found in the United States and other developed countries. Identification of the type of GBS that a patient may have can be made by electrical conductivity studies of the peripheral nerves. Other subtypes of GBS may be diagnosed based on classical symptoms of known subtypes and the location of where symptoms are experienced in the body. These variants of GBS are discussed in chapter 2.

Sudden Upsets and Unknowns

Although there is no known cure for GBS, it is reported that most patients have complete recovery over a period of weeks up to several years. Yet GBS is a serious medical problem because, approximately, up to 5% of cases can be fatal, and as much as 10% of victims can have some sort of permanent disability. Also, due to the acute onset, GBS can have an emotionally devastating impact on the family. In general, it appears that the shorter the duration of symptoms, the better the outcome. The GBS patient may suddenly be unable to work for an unknown period of time. Other members of the family will have upset routines while needing to provide support to the GBS patient undergoing diagnosis, treatment, and therapy.

This book is intended to give the GBS patient, his or her family members, and other support people the basic knowledge about an uncommon medical condition that can suddenly impact the normal course of life overnight. By understanding what is going on during this malfunction of the immune system and by knowing what is available for conventional treatments, the patient is better able to make informed decisions along with attending physicians. Also, in knowing of the cutting-edge research being done on GBS, the patient takes a more active role in understanding what is going on inside his or her body. Finally, and most importantly, this book takes the GBS patient beyond the realm of a wait-and-see approach during recovery to becoming directly involved in promoting the healing process. Research studies provide abundant evidence that many inflammatory conditions such as GBS have the potential of being improved simply by eating foods that are highly concentrated in antioxidants and other nutraceuticals (i.e., natural food chemicals and supplements that have protective and healing abilities). This book lists the best "Superfoods" and supplements for this purpose based on the most recent research findings. This book also differs from other books on GBS by giving techniques for breathing practices, referred to as Breath Work, which has also been shown to lessen inflammation and stress. It is hoped that this book will impress upon its readers that the GBS patient has the potential to take a role in controlling the unknown in GBS by using these ways for an optimum recovery.

CHAPTER 2

Diagnosing Guillain-Barré Syndrome

Early Signs

P RELIMINARY DIAGNOSIS OF GBS may be based on observation of early paresthesias such as tingling, numbness, cramping, and pain in the extremities. Weakness in the hands or feet that comes on suddenly and progresses in a descending manner down the body or in an ascending manner up the body symmetrically (on both sides) is a characteristic of GBS. In addition, the loss of long tendon reflexes (*areflexia*) is usually checked by the doctor simply by tapping at the proper areas of the knees, arms, and ankles. If these two symptoms are confirmed, GBS may be diagnosed. However, in some cases, reflex loss may not be found in the earliest stages, so the doctor may check again a short time later. Although distinguishing features of GBS, they may not all be present in the rarer variant subtypes of GBS such as Miller Fisher syndrome, where the nerves to the head and neck are affected, and acute weakness of eye muscles, loss of balance, loss of coordination, and loss of reflexes are symptoms that are initially observed.

Testing

If breathing is affected, an electrocardiogram may be performed to rule out heart problems if blood pressure and heart rate are abnormal. A defining test for GBS, nerve conduction studies (NCS) can confirm diagnosis. Specific nerves in areas of the body affected by GBS are given small electrical shocks, and the time it takes for the electrical shock to travel and the magnitude of the shock response are measured. If it is found that the velocity of shock transmission is less than normal, this is an indication of AIDP, the demyelinating type of GBS. The axonal GBS type can be distinguished from the demyelinating AIDP, but both axonal degeneration and demyelination may be observed simultaneously.

If additional evidence is required because the medical evaluation has turned up ambiguous results, a cerebral spinal tap may be ordered. In this test, a sample of the cerebral spinal fluid bathing the spinal nerves is extracted by a long needle, which is inserted into the lumbar region of the back and tested. In almost all cases of GBS, an above-normal protein level is observed in the cerebral spinal fluid without an abnormal increase in white blood cell counts. Again, although this test result is very specific to GBS, the physician must be aware that protein levels may not be elevated in the very early stages of GBS, and this test may need to be repeated if GBS cannot be confirmed otherwise. Specific antibody blood tests may help to identify GBS, but they can be expensive. They currently take longer than nerve conduction tests, and they may not be necessary.

Type and Subtype Identification

GBS patients clinically present with a variety of symptoms and affected areas of the body. The most common types and subtypes of GBS are described here, though other rarer variants are reported. It will be helpful to be familiar with these when reading about recent research findings presented in chapters 4 and 5.

Acute Inflammatory Demyelinating Polyneuropathy (AIDP)

AIDP is reportedly the most common type of GBS found in Europe, North America, and other developed countries, and it is the leading cause of acute paralysis there. Acute symptoms include weakness of the limbs with paresthesias such as tingling, prickling, numbness, and pain progressing symmetrically and in an ascending or descending fashion. Difficulty in breathing may occur due to weakness of muscles to the diaphragm. As named, the primary damage is to the myelin sheath, which is the insulating layer of the peripheral nerves. This leads to a leaking of the electrical signal carried by the axons. Axonal damage can also occur with AIDP.

Acute Motor Axonal Neuropathy (AMAN) and Acute Motor Sensory Axonal Neuropathy (AMSAN)

These types are found to be more common in developing countries with AIDP still being the most prevalent GBS type worldwide. Both

AMAN and AMSAN exhibit acute symptoms of limb weakness but with sensory symptoms such as tingling, numbness, and pain as characteristic of AMSAN, not AMAN. Nerve damage is primarily to the nerve axons, not the myelin sheath, although AIDP may occur secondarily. These GBS types are considered to be the most difficult for recovery with axonal damage more resistant to complete regeneration. Nerve conduction studies can distinguish AMAN from AMSAN by evaluating the motor nerve and the sensory nerve responses.

Miller Fisher Syndrome (MFS)

Acute symptoms of MFS include weakness of muscles to the head, such as eyes, tongue, throat, smell, loss of reflexes, and loss of coordination and balance (*ataxia*). A person with MFS may exhibit droopy eyelids (*ptosis*) and experience double vision (*diplopia*) due to weakness of the muscles surrounding the eyes. With the additional problems of loss of balance and coordination, walking is especially difficult even though the leg muscles may not be directly affected. Recent clinical case studies report that slurred speech and difficulty in swallowing may be the earliest outward signs of MFS.

The primary site of nerve damage is uncertain in MFS as nerve conduction studies may be inconclusive. Because facial muscles may become flaccid, this GBS subtype can be mistaken for Bell's palsy; however, diminished long tendon reflexes may lead to diagnosis of GBS, especially if the patient reports having had an infection within the past couple of weeks. Symptoms usually resolve within a few months, and although this is a less common variant of GBS, the acute onset of loss of speech, inability to move the eyes or to swallow food in the most advanced cases can be quite frightening to the patient and family.

Bulbar GBS Syndrome

The Bulbar subtype is a rarer variant of GBS. It is characterized by weakness beginning in the face and throat muscles, affecting the ability to swallow and speak. Its symptoms differ from the symptoms of MFS in that eye muscle weakness and motor muscle coordination are not typical symptoms. Nerves to the diaphragm are often affected so that breathing assistance is required. As with MFS, an initial misdiagnosis of Bell's palsy may be made in the onset of Bulbar GBS, but flaccid facial muscles usually occur only on one side in Bell's palsy while in Bulbar GBS, they may start on one side and, within a short period of time, affect both sides of the face symmetrically. In Bulbar GBS, muscular weakness can descend to the hands and feet. Again, diagnosis of GBS may be made if there is also a loss of long tendon reflexes.

CHAPTER 3

Conventional Treatments

An Overview of the Approach to Treatment

ALTHOUGH THERE IS no known cure for GBS at this time, researchers are honing in on the complicated pathways of the autoimmune response involved in GBS in hopes of finding one. Conventional medical care is basically aimed at supporting the patient, allowing the body to heal on its own. Respiratory function of the patient is watched closely in case ventilation is required.

Two types of blood exchanges, generally referred to as immunotherapy, may be given in more serious cases as GBS progresses, such as if the patient becomes unable to walk. The irony is that although there is evidence that immunotherapy may improve recovery if given early enough, there are serious risks, such as blood clots or infections, involved in these procedures, so the physician may wait to observe the progression of symptoms. Drugs may be given in attempts to lessen pain. Physical therapy is prescribed for regaining muscular strength, for coordination, and for fatigue as soon as possible. The patient may then be observed for a period of a few months to several years, depending on the length of time to recover.

Breathing Assistance

If the GBS patient is having difficulty breathing, evaluating the potential need for breathing assistance is of utmost importance. Positive pressure ventilation (PPV) may be administered for breathing that is noticeably weakened. If the patient has not identified difficulty in breathing, a rapid heart rate and low blood levels of oxygen may still indicate labored breathing. Another indication for the need of breathing assistance is when the patient is being treated for another existing condition, such as cardiovascular disease. In the event that GBS is progressing rapidly or if the throat muscles are involved, admittance to the intensive care unit of the hospital for patient observation may be recommended just in case breathing assistance becomes necessary.

Immunotherapy

There are two types of immunotherapy treatments that have been shown to be effective in shortening the duration of GBS: *Plasmapheresis* and high-dose *intravenous immunoglobulin* (IVIg) immunotherapies have been found to be most effective if administered within two weeks of diagnosis. Within this time frame, immunotherapy treatment may alleviate the duration of GBS symptoms in some cases, but it does not eliminate them. They may not be appropriate for mild cases, where the patient is likely to recover completely without treatment, because there are some risks involved with immunotherapy.

Plasmapheresis attempts to reverse the autoimmune response by filtering out the antibodies, which are in the plasma fraction of the blood. The remaining fraction of the patient's blood consisting of blood cells along with plasma from a donor is then pumped back into the body. This procedure is usually done five times, requiring approximately two hours each time.

In IVIg therapy, the patient is injected with relatively large amounts of donor immunoglobulin (Ig) that is matched to the patient's antibody type. This procedure appears to help by apparently blocking the inflammatory autoimmune response. The advantage of IVIg is that it is less invasive than plasmapheresis, not requiring a large catheter, it is less expensive, and it is reported to be possibly more effective. A course of treatment involves five treatments on five consecutive days.

Medications

Because the GBS patient may be sedentary for long periods of time, blood thinners may be prescribed to prevent blood clots. Medications may also be given to lessen pain with antidepressants initially prescribed for this purpose. Nonsteroidal anti-inflammatory drugs (NSAIDS)—including aspirin, ibuprofen, acetaminophen, and others—are also commonly given to minimize pain. Though they may not be completely effective, they are safer than narcotics, such as codeine, which are often combined with NSAIDS. Narcotics can lower respiration, a potentially dangerous situation in GBS patients who may already be experiencing breathing difficulty. Despite the fact that corticosteroids have no evidence of being effective and that they are well-known to cause serious side effects, they continue to be prescribed as a common conventional treatment for pain and inflammation. It is up to the patient to decide if he would rather cope with pain that does not appear to be a cardiovascular risk, but this must be done in consultation with the attending physician.

Rehabilitation

Long-term follow-up using physical therapy is important to regain muscular strength and coordination once the patient is able. It is recommended that physical therapy begin shortly after the acute phase, usually within four weeks, even though pain may persist with improvement most noticeable at the beginning and becoming more gradual, possibly up to several years.

The purpose of rehabilitation is to return the patient to his normal life as it was before acquiring GBS in as much as is possible. Programs are customized by teams to develop muscular strength and normal body functioning during the recovery period, which cannot be predicted with any great certainty. Occupational therapists may be involved in attempts to return the patient to his former employment. Coordination of transportation must be made for physical therapy that needs to be performed at special facilities away from home and in the home environment where support may be needed by the patient until he reaches a certain level of independence. Social workers assist in providing available resources to help the patient and his family make decisions to best fit their needs and transition through what may be a lengthy recovery process.

PART II

Guillain-Barré Syndrome and Cutting-Edge Research

CHAPTER 4

Latest Findings in Causes, Diagnoses, and Prognoses

Research Brings Hope

THERE IS A tremendous amount of research effort being given to all autoimmune disorders, including arthritis, asthma, diabetes, cardiovascular disease, inflammatory bowel syndrome, food allergies, and neuropathies such as multiple sclerosis and GBS. In discovering the specific course of events that occur during the body's attack on its own nervous system in GBS, future treatments may improve outcomes by shortening the duration and severity of symptoms. Some investigations are even looking at the possibility of developing vaccines to prevent the occurrence of GBS in the first case. Also, ongoing research may show ways to improve the body's natural healing process in an autoimmune attack such as by promoting nerve regeneration in GBS.

Relatives, friends, and other support people are constantly searching for the most up-to-date information about the causes, diagnoses, and prognoses of this affliction that suddenly impacts the lives of the GBS victim. They want to know as much as possible about this mysterious medical problem so that they can make the best possible decisions for getting better. To help meet this need for the most up-to-date information, the latest findings in medical science reports about causes, diagnoses, and prognoses were reviewed.

Only the most recent and relevant discoveries are summarized here, gleaning information from hundreds and hundreds of professionally recognized peer-reviewed research papers. Best efforts have been made to convert what is typically very technical medical literature into terms that can be easily understood by the general public although it is necessary to maintain a degree of technicality in order to relay the significant breaking news about GBS.

Latest Findings in Causes

The most commonly identified cause of axonal GBS is a recent infection from the bacterium *Campylobacter jejuni* (*C. jejuni*), which causes gastrointestinal problems. In industrialized countries, *C. jejuni* infections appear to be mostly associated with poultry while in developing countries, they seem to be tied to contaminated drinking water. When questioned, many GBS patients will recall having had a gastrointestinal episode or other infection within the past couple of weeks; however, doctors will usually not test for specific prior infections as they focus on testing to confirm GBS and making decisions about how to proceed with treatment of the patient, which must take priority. Other inflammatory conditions have been found to trigger GBS, including inflammatory bowel disease and even surgery.

- In axonal types of GBS (AMAN, AMSAN), prior recent infections from or exposure to *Helicobacter pylori* (*H. pylori*) or *Campylobacter jejuni* (*C. jejuni*) have been found to be associated with GBS. Other recent infections such as flu, pneumonia, hepatitis, and parvovirus have also been linked to the development of GBS within a short period of time.
- The third recurring episode of GBS was reported in a nine-year-old girl with celiac disease. The author points out that molecular mimicry involved in the allergic response to gluten may also trigger GBS.
- A 2011 research report is the first to give proof that molecular mimicry causes the autoimmune response in GBS. In this study, animals were injected with human antibodies to *C. jejuni*, and they were found to develop GBS.
- An unusually high frequency of AMAN GBS (67%) was found to be associated with a preceding *C. jejuni* infection, leading to 14% mortality and 29% severe disabilities in a controlled study of one hundred participants.
- Scientists have identified specific antibodies in GBS patients to glycosides associated with a preceding heat stable strain of a *C. jejuni* infection.
- A study on the contamination of chicken parts randomly chosen from grocery stores in Baltimore, Maryland, showed a high correlation between *C. jejuni* strains isolated from the raw meat

to those identified in axonal GBS patients. This indicates a high possibility of contracting GBS from improper handling and cooking of raw poultry.

- In a study of mice modeling GBS, it has been discovered that there is an apparent genetic risk factor in its development. Also, more recently, a report on research on Chinese patients gives evidence of a greater genetic risk for developing the AMAN and AMSAN types of GBS due to pro-inflammatory cytokines of a specific genotype.
- Although the 1976 swine flu (H1N1) vaccine reportedly caused an increase in GBS, according to the US Center for Disease Control (CDC), data indicate no statistically *significant* difference between H1N1 and other seasonal flu vaccinations in developing GBS. A 2009 CDC study reports that benefits of the flu vaccine far outweigh the risk of GBS.
- Also, a Dutch study found no significant correlation to recurring GBS symptoms and flu vaccines after years of diagnosis of GBS.

Latest Findings in Diagnosis and Prognosis

It is important to have a systematic approach to diagnosis. There are other medical conditions that may initially appear to be causing symptoms elicited by GBS. Nutritional deficiencies, diabetes, and hypothyroidism are more common than GBS, and they can also cause weakness and numbness in peripheral nerves. On the other hand, a GBS victim may not seek immediate medical attention because symptoms may appear to be flu-like or that they are a result of overexertion.

The sooner the diagnosis, the earlier the treatment can begin if deemed necessary by the attending physicians. In some milder cases, it may be recommended to just allow the patient to spontaneously recover while being observed because there are some risks involved with treatments. However, in more serious cases, the sooner the treatments are begun, the extent of damage to the nervous system is likely to be lessened, and the prognosis for complete recovery is better. That is why it is so important for the medical community to be aware of the hallmark symptoms of GBS and to begin diagnostic testing as soon as possible. By simply testing reflex responses, the physician may obtain very early indications of GBS.

As explained in chapter 2, nerve conduction studies can help diagnose GBS. If necessary, a spinal tap check of the cerebral spinal fluid can help to clarify the patient's condition. Although testing for serum antibodies may lend support to diagnosing GBS, a research report points out that motor and sensory nerve conduction tests may save several days in diagnosis, allowing treatment to begin sooner. While it is impossible to include all the breaking news in GBS research here, the following discoveries may be of interest to the reader who wants to know as much as possible about this condition:

- *Hyperreflexia*, in which reflex responses are greater than normal, have been observed in axonal GBS. The authors of this report state that this is important for physicians to be aware of this finding observed in other cases since the two main ways used to diagnose GBS are symptoms of progressive motor weakness in addition to areflexia, loss of tendon reflexes.
- In a case study, a patient was experiencing numbness around the mouth with difficulty breathing and speaking. The significance of this report is that nasalized speech, which comes on suddenly, especially following a recent infection, should be recognized by experts as an early marker of a variant of GBS. Interestingly, in another study, this oropharyngeal variant of GBS (Bulbar GBS) was confirmed in a sixteen-year-old girl who had experienced watery diarrhea two days prior to developing a nasal voice and loss of muscle control in her palate. This study also concludes that sudden onset of a nasalized speech is an early marker of GBS to direct testing for early identification with nerve conduction studies, so treatment can begin while other confirmatory tests may be pending.
- A study by the Department of Neurology in India reports that although all AMAN-type GBS patients experienced hand weakness, finger drop was the predominant symptom that was observed. In these cases, patients had normal strength in flexing fingers toward their palms but not in lifting or extending fingers outward. This study concludes that finger drop should be used as an early warning sign of the AMAN GBS subtype.
- A GBS patient who had improved with IVIg therapy and was released from the hospital had developed severe pain in his left arm within a short period of time thereafter. He was treated with a second IVIg, which gave no improvement. Further tests showed severe neuropathy of the radial nerve of the left arm only. The patient later mentioned that his wife usually slept with her head

on his left arm, which led the authors to report on the danger of nerve compression in GBS patients, leading to further nerve degeneration. This study indicates that pressure on an area of the body affected by GBS may not only delay recovery but possibly cause further degeneration by restricting blood flow.

- A study of GBS patient outcome was found to be associated with total immunoglobulin serum levels measured two weeks after receiving IVIg therapy. Although all patients had been given the same dose per body weight, circulating immunoglobulin levels varied widely. Specifically, patients having low Delta IgG levels recovered significantly more slowly, and fewer could walk after six months. The researchers conclude that those GBS patients with only a small increase in IgG levels following the first course of IVIg may benefit from an immediate second course.

- The US Center for Disease Prevention and Control (CDC) reports that although poliovirus has largely been controlled worldwide, developing nations still seem to focus on poliovirus as the cause of acute flaccid paralysis instead of GBS. The CDC found that subjects in Guatemala who had previously reported acute weakness and paralysis were evaluated with a focus on poliovirus. Patients' symptoms were dismissed when the poliovirus was not confirmed, and they were sent home even though there are obvious differences between these two medical conditions. The implication is that GBS may be much more prevalent worldwide than reported and that a systematic approach to diagnosing GBS in developing countries is urgently needed.

Again, according to these reports, awareness of the symptoms at the onset of GBS by medical professionals is critical to early diagnosis and optimum patient outcome. Developing countries are in particular need of educating the medical community to this most common cause of acute onset paralysis.

CHAPTER 5

Recent Research Studies of Conventional Treatments

Effectiveness

THE FOLLOWING RECENT research reports evaluate the effectiveness of the most common conventional treatments for GBS:

- Intravenous immunoglobulin (IVIg) therapy appears to be the treatment of choice for GBS. Because IVIg treatments are given off-label (that is, use of a drug or therapy for conditions not specifically approved), such as for neuropathies, the American Association of Neuromuscular and Electrodiagnostic Medicine (AANEM) formed an ad hoc committee to review medical literature reports of the effectiveness of IVIg although it had been used for over twenty years for various neuromuscular conditions. The AANEM ad hoc committee developed a scale-rating medical support for specific neuropathies with categories ranging from class I to class IV, with class I having enough evidence in the medical literature to support its use. GBS was rated class I, very effective.
- It is reported that most GBS patients improve with IVIg therapy, though some may not respond as well and GBS symptoms may continue to worsen. As mentioned in chapter 4, a research report supports performing a second IVIg in GBS patients where blood serum levels show only a small increase shortly following the first IVIg injection.
- An update report on GBS gives information that large randomized trials have shown both IVIg and plasma exchange to be effective treatments but that corticosteroids have not been successful in lessening symptoms. In a 2010 study done of GBS patient outcomes following four weeks of oral corticosteroid use, there

were significantly less improvements than those who had not taken steroids. It was found that not only did steroids delay recovery but that the drug also appeared to be associated with significantly more diabetes cases requiring insulin.

Cutting-Edge Research

There is much ongoing research investigating specific components of the immune system as it becomes involved in the cascading events of a very complicated autoimmune response in GBS. Due to the extremely technical nature of this medical literature, detailed findings are summarized, where necessary, for the broad audience of this book. Many technical references are provided at the back of this book for those who want to read about this exciting area of medical research. This area of GBS research is extremely important since targeting the immune system may likely be the future key to controlling the runaway autoimmune response in GBS.

- A research group reports the possibility of treating GBS patients with anti-antibodies to neutralize the antibodies that attack molecules found on healthy human nerves.
- Research aimed at prevention of GBS from *C. jejuni* infection studied the susceptibility of this bacterium to antibiotics. The bacterium *C. jejuni* has a reputation of being antibiotic resistant; however, this study identifies those which have been found to be effective in killing *C. jejuni*. There is particular interest in inhibiting *C. jejuni* in Japan, where this organism is associated with the development of GBS more than any other known cause.

News in Rehabilitation Therapy

- In looking at rehabilitation of GBS patients, studies indicate that long-term follow-up by medical professionals after one year of diagnosis is very important. One study found that persistent pain and difficulty in walking were still common after one year and that the patient should be informed to have reasonable expectations for a long period of recovery.
- Studies show that most of the improvement process occurs within the first six months following GBS onset. After one year of diagnosis, most of the disruption to normal life was found to

be a lack of a sense of well-being and decreased social activities due to muscle aches and cramps as scored by GBS patients in a standardized survey and not due to depression.

- A rehabilitation study by the Department of Neurology at the University Medical Center in the Netherlands reported that many neuromuscular disorders can cause peripheral fatigue, but with GBS, fatigue is not necessarily related to the severity of this condition, and it can become long lasting. This report states that although fatigue may be an initial defense for the body by inducing rest during the acute onset phase, recommendations are to begin exercise as therapy for fatigue immediately following treatment for other GBS symptoms.

CHAPTER 6

Breaking News in Natural Anti-inflammatories

A Search for Complementary Therapies

A REVIEW OF CURRENT publications in relation to the use of complementary therapies for GBS—that is, therapies that are used by physicians along with conventional medical care—revealed little information. Reports regarding the potential effectiveness of acupuncture indicate a need for further research in this area:

- In a clinical report of a seventeen-year-old girl who had been diagnosed with chronic inflammatory demyelinating polyneuropathy—a peripheral neuropathy similar to the AIDP type of GBS but which is recurring—acupuncture treatment was successful.
- The potential treatment of GBS using electroacupuncture at specific nerve locations in GBS animal models has been studied. It was found that nerve conduction measurements showed significant improvement along the sciatic nerve with electroacupuncture as compared to those without the treatment.

Controlled research studies in the application of complementary and natural therapies are urgently needed, especially considering that there can be extended periods of recovery during which debilitating weakness, pain, and other symptoms may linger for months or years.

One of the purposes of this book is to help GBS patients help themselves to optimize their recovery. Due to the paucity of research studies being reported in complementary and natural therapies for GBS, non-GBS specific areas of research relating to inflammation and the autoimmune response were investigated. The most relevant evidence-based breaking news in natural ways to control inflammation is presented here. It is exciting to know that simple means such as anti-inflammatory foods and supplements, light therapy, breathing exercises, and restful sleep can play an important role in aiding the GBS patient's recovery because this information empowers the GBS patient to take a role in promoting healing. The following studies support the use of these natural anti-inflammatories:

Anti-inflammatory Omega-3 Fatty Acids

- Fish oil and other omega-3 dietary sources are well recognized for their anti-inflammatory effects. Researchers believe that our typical contemporary Western diets have become highly unbalanced in the two main types of fatty acids we ingest and that this has led to many health problems. It is thought that humans in general consumed much more omega-3 fatty acids even just a few centuries ago. Our ancestors' diets might have contained a ratio of 1:1 of omega-6 fatty acids to omega-3 fatty acids. Today, it is estimated to be in a ratio of 10 to 20:1 omega-6 to omega-3 fatty acids. Because omega-6 fatty acids are pro-inflammatory and omega-3 fatty acids are anti-inflammatory, this imbalance may be a major contributor to obesity and metabolic syndrome, which includes biomarkers of inflammation, such as insulin resistance and high levels of C-reactive protein (CRP) and heart disease.
- Lifestyle intervention of metabolic syndrome patients looked at how diet and exercise affected inflammation and insulin resistance. In this evaluation of six studies, it was shown that improvements in dietary composition and exercise consistently showed improvements and that a healthy diet was even more effective than exercise in reducing inflammation and insulin resistance.
- Consistent evidence from a study on the effect of omega-3 fatty acids on the health of the retina indicates that omega-3s have a protective effect against inflammation and oxidation that lead to diseases of the retina.

Despite the fact that experts believe that this dietary change in the types of fats we eat over the past relatively short period of time could be the single most important contributor to inflammatory diseases, there is little emphasis on this for disease prevention:

- A research report from Belgium states that although recommendations have been established for school lunch programs, hospitals, and the general population for the most part, they have not changed to a healthy balance of foods containing omega-3s. The report goes on to state that even during the first year of life, babies are mostly being fed commercial foods containing omega-6 fatty acids to supplement their milk, far different from the dietary guidelines. It would appear that the medical community could take a larger role in educating the public in the importance of eating foods high in omega-3 fatty acids, therefore being proactive in helping to prevent chronic diseases believed to be caused by inflammation.

Protective Herbs, Spices, and Food Chemicals

Anti-inflammatory extracts are reviewed in a paper about Eastern Mediterranean plants. Reasons for the effectiveness of folk remedies are given, explaining that water extracts of herbs have been shown to contain chemicals such as phenols, alkaloids, glycosides, and carbohydrates, chemicals for which scientific evidence shows anti-inflammatory properties.

Breaking news in natural anti-inflammatories continues to provide evidence that foods work to keep us healthy:

- Many studies have shown Mediterranean herbs to be highly antioxidant.
- The spice turmeric was investigated to determine how the active antioxidant component curcumin, a polyphenol, may work in the body since it has been reported to be a powerful antiarthritic. It was found that curcumin inhibits inflammatory pathways in osteoarthritis by inhibiting cartilage degradation.
- An extract of black rice was found to be a powerful antioxidant contributing to the lowering of biomarkers for atherosclerosis in mice. It is thought that anthocyanins in the black rice act as the antioxidants.
- The protective effects of bilberry—another anthocyanin found in dark blue and purple fruits, such as blueberries—were studied in mice serving as models for cardiovascular disease. Amazingly, it was found that after only two weeks of supplementing bilberry, genes

responsible for liver inflammation decreased and cholesterol uptake markedly improved.

- The health benefits of drinking red wine (in moderation) is primarily attributed to the antioxidant resveratrol. A research study on the effects of resveratrol in the body showed that this natural compound found in red grapes blocked the pathway leading to inflammation. Specifically, it inhibited transcription of the genes that cause inflammation by interferon-activated macrophages.

Anti-inflammatory Properties of Vitamin D3

Vitamin D3 has been shown to help regulate the immune responses. Recently, vitamin D3 has been the "new" vitamin of interest with concerns that the general population may not be getting enough of this vitamin. Interestingly, although a government advisory council reports that the average US diet is not deficient in vitamin D3, the Recommended Daily Allowances, however, have been increased from 400 IU units of supplementation to 600 IU for ages one to seventy years old and to 800 IU for those over seventy.

Indeed, research shows a link between low levels of vitamin D3 and disease. Breaking news research on the connection between vitamin D3 and inflammation, therefore, was investigated for the purpose of this book to see if there is any evidence that supplementing with this vitamin may be helpful to the GBS patient. The following studies support the anti-inflammatory role of vitamin D3 in the role of atherosclerosis and proper immune function for disease control:

- Since it is known that dendritic cells of neurons modulate the immune response through T cells, researchers looked at these immunoregulatory capabilities of vitamin D3. They discovered that vitamin D3 generated T cell immune suppressors, which would decrease the immune response. Scientists suggest that anti-inflammatory drugs containing vitamin D3 could have the potential to treat many chronic inflammatory conditions.
- Other studies have looked at the anti-inflammatory effects of vitamin D in cardiovascular disease, finding evidence for the potential of therapeutically supplementing with this vitamin.
- A laboratory in the Netherlands studied the seasonal variation of the immune response in the body. It is well-known that the human

body can synthesize vitamin D3 when the skin is exposed to sunlight, and the Netherlands receives very little sunlight for much of the year due to its high northern latitudes. With less vitamin D3 being produced during days of little sunlight, researchers found higher measurements of inflammatory biomarkers as compared to days of more sunlight. From this study, it can be inferred that vitamin D3 levels were relatively low during days of longer darkness, and that is why measurements for inflammation were higher.

Alpha-lipoic Acid (ALA)

Two of the more familiar antioxidants required for proper functioning of the body are vitamins C and E, and there have been many studies on their anti-inflammatory and protective properties. Some antioxidants are not as familiar, but they are extremely important in supporting the endogenous antioxidant network. Alpha-lipoic acid, an amino acid, is one of these:

Alpha-lipoic acid is an antioxidant that also plays an important role in energy production. It is an amino acid that is made in the body, and since it is both fat and water soluble, it is found in all parts of our cells. Alpha-lipoic acid has been used for over thirty years in Germany to slow neuropathy in diabetics. Its properties are also being investigated for its potential role in helping cardiovascular disease, hypertension, inflammation, cancer, and in the treatment of Alzheimer's disease.

Making a Difference Naturally

These breaking news reports provide scientific evidence of the role that foods can play in keeping inflammation under control. Controlled studies of the antioxidants in foods are just beginning to elucidate how they keep our bodies operating in a balanced state of health. It should be no surprise that whole, unprocessed, naturally-occurring foods act as preventative medicine in the body. After all, these kinds of foods are what the body was intended to use for fuel and upkeep.

As a GBS patient, any changes to your routine should be approved by your physician prior to implementation, but by switching to an anti-inflammatory diet, science shows that you have the potential to help your body make the repairs necessary for recovery. Chapter 8 explains how antioxidants in foods and supplements help to control inflammation. Chapter 10 lists antioxidant-rich Superfoods to help guide you in planning the must-haves in your new anti-inflammatory diet. Additionally, "Super Mood Foods" are included in the appendix for ready-to-go anti-inflammatory menus to fit your mood of the day.

The essence of this book is to present evidence-based, safe, and natural anti-inflammatory therapies that, with your doctor's approval, can be used to complement conventional medical care. The recovery process in GBS can be frustratingly and agonizingly slow. As you read further here, you will learn of another evidence-based natural therapy for inflammation, *Breath Work*, which can be incorporated as an essential daily routine. By taking an active role in recovery by eating Superfoods, taking supplements, and practicing Breath Work, the GBS patient has the potential to make a real impact on the healing process. *Please note that it is important to always obtain the approval of your physician prior to implementing any changes to your diet or routine to ensure that they do not interfere with your regular medical care.*

PART III

Controlling Inflammation: The Key to Recovery

CHAPTER 7

Why Inflammation Causes Damage

What is Inflammation?

AS A PART of our everyday normal functioning, inflammation protects the body from foreign invaders such as bacteria, viruses, and cancer cells attempting to get established. Inflammation also plays a role in wound healing, where white blood cells help to remove damaged cells and signal the production of new replacement cells. Inflammation is necessary for survival.

Acute inflammation is characterized by a rapid onset of symptoms—such as redness, swelling, pain, increased blood flow, and infiltration of white blood cells—lasting for only several days and up to four to six weeks. This may occur as a normal response as in an infection or an injury, but unfortunately, acute inflammation may occur as an autoimmune response as in GBS. Chronic inflammation, as opposed to acute, is long lasting. Scientists now know that chronic inflammation can lead to heart disease, diabetes, arthritis, asthma, inflammatory bowel disease, and many other chronic and serious conditions.

Inflammation in GBS

Symptoms of acute onset of GBS typically appear within a period of a few days and up to two weeks after a triggering event. Scientists have found evidence that in GBS, the trigger, which may be a virus or bacteria, initiates an autoimmune response where the body mistakenly signals an attack on healthy nerve roots, the myelin sheath, the axons, or a combination of these sites. Inflammatory white blood cells called leukocytes signal the release of highly reactive *free radicals* in this process. Normal nerve transmission is disrupted as the myelin sheath is damaged in the AIDP subtype of GBS or when the axons are directly attacked as in the AMAN or AMSAN GBS subtype.

The result of inflammation of the peripheral nerves may lead to the GBS symptoms of weakness, pain, tingling sensation, and the eventual loss of motor control of the limbs and head. When inflammation causes damage to the nerves that control the diaphragm, the patient may require hospitalization and breathing assistance. Internal organs such as the kidneys and intestines may also become affected and may not function properly if inflammation spreads to the autonomic nerves. A flood of inflammatory molecules are directed to the nerve surfaces, where they block nerve transmission and cause nerve degeneration. As inflammation continues, other pro-inflammatory molecules become involved, and macrophages move in to remove the "debris" of degeneration. *That is why controlling inflammation is the key to recovery in GBS.*

Antioxidants Stop Free Radical Damage

Inflammation causes the release of free radicals in the body. *Free radicals* are chemical compounds or elements that contain an extra electron, and they are highly reactive because they will release that extra electron to anything they come in contact with, causing cellular and DNA damage unless they are kept in check by the body's natural endogenous antioxidants circulating in the blood. Excess free radicals—those that exceed the quenching capacity of our endogenous antioxidants working within our bodies—have been shown to be involved in the aging process, coronary artery disease, diabetes, and other chronic diseases and conditions.

Antioxidants help to normalize the immune system, providing protection during regular body processes, such as metabolism and respiration, but they are especially important in keeping inflammation under control during infections, injury, or other stresses to the body. Antioxidants include familiar vitamins such as C and E and omega-3 fatty acids, but there are many others in the antioxidant network that work synergistically within our bodies. Also, whole healthy foods contain powerful antioxidant compounds and chemicals, which we need to eat on a regular basis to keep inflammation in check. During runaway inflammation and times of chronic stress, these antioxidants are rapidly used up and our bodies become overwhelmed by damaging free radicals.

CHAPTER 8

The Power of Antioxidants

Oxidative Stress

WHEN FREE RADICALS are formed in excess of the body's ability to neutralize them, a condition referred to as *oxidative stress* occurs. Unless oxidative stress is quickly brought under control, inflammation leading to pain, disease, and tissue damage takes place. Under normal circumstances, free radicals are kept under control by antioxidants taken into the body through foods and supplements and by antioxidants that are manufactured within the body. One of the ways that free radicals are pro-inflammatory is by directly activating genes to make components of the immune response, such as interleukin-1 (IL-1) and interleukin-6 (IL-6). When runaway inflammation occurs during an autoimmune response, it is urgent to quench the flood of free radicals as much as possible and as soon as possible in order to minimize damage to healthy cells and tissue.

Studies continue to show that oxidative stress is involved in inflammatory pain and neuropathy of diabetes, fibromyalgia, and in a simulated GBS autoimmune neuritis. Oxidative stress has also been shown to cause demyelination and degeneration in animal models. Free radicals include reactive oxygen species and reactive nitrogen species, which have been shown to be directly involved in the peripheral neuropathy of GBS.

The Role of Antioxidants in GBS Recovery

Scientists are heatedly investigating the autoimmune response at every stage of the extremely complex cascade of events leading up to inflammation with the goal to halt GBS in its tracks one day. Meanwhile, one of the simplest ways to reduce free radicals in our bodies is to increase antioxidants in our diet through foods and supplements.

Part 4 of this book concisely explains the types of foods that should become complete meals. They should become the mainstay of an anti-inflammatory diet, not merely eaten as supplements or tokens along with the same old unhealthy foods traditionally eaten. Scientific studies continue to show that endogenous antioxidant blood levels in patients with inflammatory conditions are typically low. Scientific evidence shows that because the GBS victim is in a state of oxidative stress, eating foods high in antioxidants in addition to taking antioxidant supplements are extremely important to recovery.

CHAPTER 9

The Power of the Breath

Breath Work

THE POWER OF the breath in controlling inflammation is undeniable. There are many names and styles for breathing exercises. Traditional breathing exercises in yoga practice are called *pranayama*, meaning "extension of the life" in Sanskrit. Some experts simply refer to controlled breathing practices as Breath Work, and that is how this book will refer to it. Next to a Superfood diet packed with antioxidants, Breath Work may be the single most important practice that the GBS recoverer can add to conventional medical care. Some background is presented in this chapter to help the reader understand why the breath, something we tend to take so much for granted, can play such a significant role in the recovery process. An advantage of Breath Work is that it can be practiced in a comfortable seated position anywhere and it requires no equipment. Procedures for several simple Breath Work practices are given in chapter 12.

Currently, controlled breathing is actually being used in many hospital settings as complementary therapy across the United States as the medical community is beginning to recognize accumulating scientific evidence for its many benefits. Everyone, including those who are not experiencing GBS, should plan to start off practice slowly, gradually building up the length of practice time and the ability to take a deep breath. It is truly amazing that studies have shown that benefits of Breath Work are not just psychological. They are also physiological, lowering blood levels of biomarkers for stress. The GBS patient is likely to experience much-needed feelings of relaxation, improved mood, and better sleep quality with just a few Breath Work practices. Studies show that benefits will become longer lasting with a consistent daily routine.

Background

In 1979, Jon Kabat-Zinn founded the Mindfulness-Based Stress Reduction Clinic (MBSR) based on results of many studies indicating that meditative-type practices could alleviate symptoms of chronic illnesses and pain. There is a variety of meditative-type practices, including yoga, tai chi, qigong, and others, but what was found to be the common link is that controlled breathing is at the core of mindfulness-based meditation. In the MBSR program, patients were trained to use slow, rhythmic, deep-breathing exercises along with meditation or other practices that focus on the breath. There have been many clinical studies of the MBSR program and reports of the effectiveness of using Breath Work in reducing stress-associated symptoms of chronic illnesses such as heart disease, psoriasis, type 2 diabetes, rheumatoid arthritis, fibromyalgia, and in pain. The MBSR program has been expanded into many clinical settings across the country, included as complementary therapy for patients recovering from surgery and chronic medical conditions.

Breath Work Reduces Inflammation

Contrary to most people's understanding, stress is a real biological phenomenon, not just psychologically "in the mind." Stress is measurable. Currently, blood serum levels of C-reactive protein (CRP) and cortisol are the most commonly measured biomarkers for stress. When the body is stressed either psychologically, for example, by uncontrollable events, or physiologically, such as through injury or disease, CRP and cortisol levels will significantly increase above normal levels. This is a signal that inflammation is ongoing, which can be measured by many other biomarkers, one of which is interleukin-6 (IL-6), a pro-inflammatory white blood cell that helps to trigger the autoimmune response.

There have been hundreds of studies on the benefits of practicing breath control. The following summaries provide the reader with a sampling of the most relevant recent research that continues to provide evidence for the effectiveness of Breath Work in controlling stress:

- In a controlled study using meditative qigong, researchers studied cancer patients and found that this practice significantly improved fatigue and mood, and the inflammatory biomarker C-reactive protein decreased.

- In heart failure patients practicing yoga and breathing exercises, there was an improvement in tolerance to exercise along with decreases in serum levels of IL-6 and CRP, markers of inflammation.
- In a randomized-controlled trial, MBSR was taught to participants with fibromyalgia, a chronic pain, fatigue, and insomnia syndrome. After the eight-week program of mindfulness meditation and yoga exercises, it was evaluated that the MBSR patients realized improvements in the symptoms of fibromyalgia.
- In a small study of mastectomy patients, four weeks of abdominal breathing led to reduced serum cortisol and anxiety and improved quality of life (as measured by a standardized questionnaire).
- A study by Columbia University reports that early research that showed evidence that the Tibetan practice of yoga, meditation, and a healthy diet leads to increased longevity and enhanced good health is due to the anti-inflammatory, anti-stress, and antioxidant effects of these practices.

The GBS recoverer can use the simple Breath Work practices given in chapter 12, though there are others that can be found through a literature search on the topic. Remember that it is important for the GBS patient to seek the approval of the attending physician prior to beginning the routine practice of Breath Work.

PART IV

You as Healer: Putting Out the Fire

CHAPTER 10

Eat Antioxidant-Rich Foods to Quench Inflammation

You Really Are What You Eat

CHANGING FROM THE typical US diet to one that is full of antioxidant-rich foods will likely improve the way one feels. Foods that are high in antioxidants are some of the healthiest foods in the world. Breaking news from scientific studies consistently report evidence for disease-preventative properties of foods. For instance, one of the more recent reports about the benefits of antioxidants was about the connection between strawberry consumption and the prevention of throat cancer. Because they fight free radicals, antioxidant-rich foods act as nutraceuticals, natural remedies for inflammation. These foods are extremely important to a healthy diet, and that is why this book refers to them as Superfoods. The GBS recoverer should strive to make a variety of Superfoods a major portion of each and every meal. Just as importantly, there are foods that are pro-inflammatory, which should be completely eliminated or at least minimized as discussed in this chapter.

As you read on here, you will discover why being healthy is not just about what we *are* eating that is making us prone to inflammation and disease; it is just as much about what we are *not* eating. If we fill ourselves up with mostly pro-inflammatory empty calories, our bodies' machineries are unable to produce the biochemicals that we need to operate properly and to have a healthy immune system. A balanced diet consisting of lean protein, healthy fats and oils, and complex carbohydrates in the form of whole grains, fruits, and vegetables is what our bodies required to utilize over the history of humankind for energy and for our protection.

The following concise general guidelines can help you redesign your eating habits for the purpose of battling inflammation. Pay special attention to the key words, "fats," "color," and "grains." Become familiar with the types of foods in the summary list at the end of this chapter and make use of ready-to-use recipes given in the appendix. Eventually, it will become automatic for you to plan your antioxidant-rich, anti-inflammatory meals. Once you begin to feel and see the benefits in addition to how deliciously healthy Superfoods can be, this lifestyle change may become permanent for you, adding to your vitality and longevity.

Replace Omega-6 Fatty Acids with Omega-3s and Omega-9s

There have been many studies on the anti-inflammatory properties of omega-3 fatty acids. It is thought that our ancestors' diets were very high in omega-3s from eating wild plant foods and the lean game they hunted. Experts believe that this has probably been the single most important change to modern-day diets. Today's diets contain excesses of omega-6 fatty acids from vegetable and palm oils and the many products made from them. The words "vegetable" and "corn oils" sound as though they should be healthy, but they contain omega-6 fatty acids that cause inflammatory interleukins to be produced in the body. Vegetable oils include corn, safflower, cottonseed, soy, peanut, and palm oils. They are added to many prepared foods and baked goods and constitute a major ingredient in most margarine. By reading food product labels, you will begin to see how very many foods have these ingredients in them. The good thing is that usually, these are processed foods, so if you avoid them and eat whole foods you are already on your way to a less inflammatory and healthier diet.

Foods high in omega-3s and other anti-inflammatory fatty acids include salmon, herring, sardines, mackerel, dark-green leafy vegetables, avocados, walnuts, and pecans. Use extra virgin olive oil (EVOO), which is the highest grade of olive oil, because it is the first to be collected from the pressing of the olives. EVOO contains more antioxidants, and it is more flavorful than subsequent pressings. Canola oil is also a healthy fat, containing mostly omega-3 fatty acids but also some omega-9 fatty acids while olive oil contains omega-9 fatty acids. *Olive oil and canola oil should be used on salads and in cooking, not vegetable oils, margarine, or butter, which cause inflammation.* Omega-9 fatty acids help to promote omega-3 fatty acids to make anti-inflammatory compounds in the body. Use EVOO on cooked vegetables, pasta, and salads. Some experts recommend the use of canola oil in high temperature or long-term cooking since heat can more easily oxidize EVOO, creating free radicals.

Minimize Saturated Fats

Dairy fats happen to be one of the tastiest fats on earth. They are also one of the most detrimental fats in the Western diet. Everything tastes delicious with butter and cheese on it. And who does not love ice cream and a glass of ice-cold whole milk? The trouble is that the Western European diet that Americans have traditionally carried on with cow's milk products playing such a huge role has been costly to our health. Dairy products are naturally high in saturated fats, and they should be eaten in small amounts and infrequently. It has been shown that calcium and other nutrients found in cow's milk can easily be obtained from other foods. In fact, much of the world's population does not eat cow's milk products, and they even lack the enzyme necessary to digest them.

Saturated fats, as found in dairy products and raised livestock, contain almost completely omega-6s while meat from wild animals are reported to contain mostly anti-inflammatory omega-3 fatty acids. Our bodies need fats, but throughout eons, humans have upset the balance of healthy fats. Agricultural practices to mass produce food to feed growing populations have artificially manipulated the fat balance of modern-day Western diets. Some places, on the other hand still incorporate large amounts of anti-inflammatory fats, such as olive oil, which is used extensively in Mediterranean cooking, along with abundant fruits and vegetables that are full of antioxidants.

The importance of eating healthy fats cannot be overstated. Scientists believe that the ever-growing trend of inflammatory diseases and allergies, asthma, and all those medical conditions ending in "-itis" may largely be due to the unhealthy Western-style diet. Pro-inflammatory interleukins made from omega-6s must be balanced by anti-inflammatory omega-3s; otherwise, chronic inflammation and an abnormal immune response is the result. Therefore, the first step in battling GBS through a change in diet is to include those healthy fats as described here.

Eat Colorful Vegetables and Fruits with Plenty of Herbs and Spices

Replace starchy white vegetables like white potatoes, peas, and corn with sweet potatoes, which are full of fiber and vitamins, and other brightly colored vegetables in addition to fruits. Herbs, spices, brightly colored fruits, and vegetables have high carotenoid content, powerful antioxidants.

Flavonoids are a very large class of naturally occurring chemicals called polyphenols found in fruits and vegetables. Flavonoids, carotenoids, and other polyphenols are naturally occurring antioxidants that the body can effectively use to keep free radicals in check. In particular, herbs and spices have high concentrations of antioxidants probably because these chemicals protect their plant cells from ultraviolet rays, which generate free radicals, since these plants are typically native to regions of high levels of sunlight.

In order to get healthy portions of vegetables, fill your plate half full of vegetables. Herbs and spices are often underused in the typical Western fare, yet they can make bland dishes taste delicious without the use of salt, a contributor of high blood pressure, and overused seasoning. Experiment and become familiar with all the wonderful flavors of herbs and spices, which are full of protective flavonoids and other anti-inflammatory chemicals. Replace typical high-caloric, bad-fat, nonnutritious desserts with fresh or cooked fruit sweetened with a little honey and sprinkled with sweet spices, such as cinnamon, nutmeg, allspice, or cardamom.

Eliminate Bad Carbohydrates

Refined sugars and other *simple* carbohydrates (think "processed," "flours," "sweet drinks") are not what our bodies were intended to digest. These could be called nonfoods, and although they provide quick energy, they are inflammatory because they do so. When blood sugar levels rapidly spike, cells cannot absorb the glucose quickly enough. Excess glucose lingers in the bloodstream, where it oxidizes, generating destructive free radicals. Glucose also reacts with proteins in the skin, such as collagen, and with tissues, such as the lens in your eyes, promoting cataracts. This process is called glycation, causing premature wrinkling and sagging skin. The rate at which the body can absorb glucose is limited. A regular diet of simple carbohydrates such as baked goods, sweets, pasta, white potatoes, and white bread can make our cells become insulin resistant, unable to absorb glucose. This leads to prediabetes, then diabetes, a very serious inflammatory, progressive, and neuropathic disease.

Type 2 diabetes is a serious disease of epic proportions now spreading worldwide. Even if someone has not reached this state of imbalance, eliminating foods that contain added sugar, corn syrup, and finely milled flours (which are just as readily absorbed into the bloodstream as sugar) is a huge step in the anti-inflammatory direction. Replacing typical desserts with fresh fruit topped with low-fat Greek yogurt and sprinkling with nuts, spices, wheat germ, or unsweetened granola can be very satisfying and nutritious. Using only whole grain breads (whole wheat is not whole grain) and eating whole grains, especially brown rice, will not only give you a welcome change to your everyday, previously limited range of foods. It will also open doors to the possibility of a whole new way of cooking.

If the GBS recoverer wishes to do everything possible to optimize his or her outcome, dietary discipline is necessary to help quench the fire of inflammation. A half cup of pasta or bread that is not whole grain is fine a couple of times a week as long as it is eaten along with a large serving of salad or plenty of vegetables because by eating foods high in fiber, the speed at which glucose is released into the bloodstream is slowed during digestion. Instead of butter or margarine, use extra virgin olive oil seasoned with herbs and garlic for dipping whole grain bread and drizzle this healthy fat onto pasta because this will also slow the absorption of carbohydrates. As a bonus, you will delight in the burst of flavor this small but significant change will give you.

Lactose Intolerance and Food Allergies

In many countries around the world, milk products are used very little or not at all, especially in the adult diet. Studies have shown that bone density does not correlate with the amount of consumption of milk products even in children. A balanced diet that includes plenty of green leafy vegetables, fish, beans, walnuts, and soybeans (edamame, tofu, tempeh, soy milk, etc.) can provide plenty of calcium to meet the body's needs. It is important to eat foods also abundant in vitamin D (e.g., eggs, fatty fish) as this vitamin is essential in assimilating calcium. Since excess sodium interferes with calcium absorption, replace salt with other seasonings and refreshing lemon zest.

Although dairy products can be very nutritious and they are supplemented with vitamin D, which studies have shown to be anti-inflammatory, many people have lactose intolerance and cannot digest milk products. Some experts argue that it is unnatural for humans to consume cow's milk, and this is the reason why so many people around the world are lacking the enzyme, lactase, to digest lactose, the sugar in cow's milk. Lactase is also sometimes lost as we age. The result is referred to as lactose intolerance, which causes the discomfort of gas and pain in the abdomen, accompanied by water being drawn into the intestines. This can occur within twenty minutes from the time of drinking milk or eating milk products, such as cheese or ice cream, and the easiest way to tell if one is lactose intolerant is to eliminate dairy products and observe if these problems go away, if they were present.

Lactose intolerance and other food sensitivities must be taken seriously. Some food allergies can cause an acute allergic response, such as a skin rash, hives, or even anaphylactic shock. People who have this problem are well aware that these reactions can occur, and they are very careful to avoid those foods that cause these reactions. Others may notice that they experience discomfort shortly after eating certain foods, but they continue to eat them because the symptoms are temporary.

Celiac disease is a serious condition caused by sensitivity to gluten, the protein found in wheat and other grains. Continuation of eating foods containing gluten can lead to a long list of medical problems, including persistent anemia and other nutritional deficiencies, internal hemorrhaging, and nervous system damage. Celiac disease is also associated with the development of many other autoimmune diseases. Reportedly, celiac disease occurs in as many as three people in one hundred.

The important point to be made here is that food allergies and sensitivities cause inflammation. Continuation of eating foods that cause this can lead to damage of the intestinal wall and a leaky gut, allowing pathogens and undigested foods to pass through. This predisposes the person to a host of other autoimmune diseases. The GBS patient should immediately speak to his or her physician about testing for any suspected food intolerance, food allergy, or food sensitivity. These foods can be rigorously avoided if there is a strong suspicion that they are causing problems because such foods cause an additional burden on the already existing inflammatory state of the GBS patient.

Superfood Summary List

The following is a list of the most common Superfoods. Although all fruits and vegetables contain vitamins, minerals, fiber, and other nutrients, those that are highly colored contain the highest levels of antioxidants with the exception of onions and garlic, which contain unique, potent sulfur-containing antioxidant chemicals. Even some fruits and vegetables—such as white potatoes, parsnips, and bananas—are very *glycemic*; that is, they contain starches and sugars that are released very quickly as glucose into the bloodstream, so they should be avoided. Yams and sweet potatoes, on the other hand, are not in the potato family, and they are an excellent source of nutrients and antioxidants, releasing glucose much more slowly than white potatoes due to their high fiber content. Because the GBS patient may have another medical condition or is taking medications where dietary restrictions are important, the physician's approval should be obtained before beginning any new dietary changes. It would be good to take along this list of Superfoods for the doctor to quickly review and to make comments on if necessary.

Fruits—Berries (blueberries, blackberries, strawberries, raspberries, etc.); red, purple, and black grapes; cherries; citrus fruits (oranges, grapefruits, tangerines, etc.); avocados; apples; watermelons; cantaloupes; and tropical fruits (e.g., kiwi, guava, mango, pineapple, and papaya)

Vegetables—Dark-green leafy vegetables, such as spinach, escarole, beet greens, dark-green and purple lettuces, and especially broccoli, bok choy, brussels sprouts, kale, collards, purple cabbage, carrots, sweet potatoes, and the much larger variety, yams, winter squash (pumpkin, butternut, acorn, etc.), and onions

Beans—Also referred to as legumes, are high in folate and antioxidants, especially lentils, black, kidney, garbanzo, lima, and soybeans in all forms, such as tofu, edamame, and low-salt soy sauce

Fish—All seafood in general is a good source of magnesium, a mineral that promotes relaxation. High concentrations of omega-3 fatty acids are found in salmon, mackerel, tuna and sardines. However, limit intake of tuna to once a week to minimize the potential accumulation of mercury in the body.

Whole Grains—Especially long grain and brown rice, quinoa and whole grain oats, barley, and wheat. Remember that "whole wheat" is not whole grain and be aware that many ready-to-eat boxed cereals are usually not whole grain; they contain added sugars, and they are typically supplemented with too much iron and other metals, all of which are pro-inflammatory.

Mushrooms—A low-calorie source of B vitamins, antioxidants, and protein. Shiitake and cremini varieties have been shown to enhance a normal immune function.

Nuts and Seeds—Especially walnuts, pecans, almonds, flax, and sesame seeds, which are full of healthy fat, lignins, and vitamin E

Herbs and Spices—Herbs, especially oregano, basil, cilantro, rosemary, and garlic; spices, especially turmeric, cumin, cinnamon, and ginger

Drinks—Tea, especially white and green, unsweetened or with sugar substitute. Avoid drinking late in the day since it contains caffeine, which is a stimulant that can interfere with sleep, so avoid drinking late in the day. Some fruit juices are loaded with antioxidants (e.g., pomegranate, concord grape, blueberry, cherry, and cranberry), but look for these without added sugar or corn syrup.

Dark Chocolate—Contains highly antioxidant flavonoids. Eat in small amounts due to high levels of saturated fats. Avoid milk chocolate, which has lower levels of antioxidants but high sugar content. Chocolate contains caffeine, so avoid eating late in the day to prevent sleep interference.

Bonus! To get you off to a running start, a variety of Super Mood Food recipes are included in the appendix of this book. These recipes range from those extremely simple to prepare to those more dinner-like; however, it is intended that they be chosen by the GBS recoverer according to what he or she feels like eating at that particular time (Super Mood Foods), not by what is typically defined as breakfast, lunch, or dinner. Eating according to one's mood will enhance the likelihood of eating what the body needs. When adding variety and balance in the types of foods included throughout the day, meal types should not matter.

Hopefully, these recipes will inspire a whole new way of preparing colorful, flavorful, antioxidant-rich Superfoods to supercharge your body for recovery from GBS and beyond and to bring you optimum health and longevity.

CHAPTER 11

Take Antioxidant
Supplements as Backup

D URING NEUROPATHIC INFLAMMATION such as with GBS, the body manufactures and overwhelms the nerves with free radicals as part of the autoimmune response. These highly reactive atoms and molecules must be neutralized as quickly as possible to prevent further tissue and DNA damage. Eating an abundance of antioxidant-rich Superfoods will go a long way toward helping your body fight inflammation, but it is probably a good idea to take supplements to ensure that you are supplying enough antioxidants to quench the flood of free radicals as quickly as possible. *Always check with your physician before beginning any new vitamin regimen plan.*

According to health experts, the following supplements are especially important. Although other antioxidants may be advocated, the body is normally able to produce them, or else they are abundant in a healthy diet. The following supplements should not be replaced by a single multivitamin, which would likely not contain the dosages as listed below. However, some supplements may be sold in a combined supplement, such as calcium and magnesium or selenium and zinc, since they are synergistic, so they are in balanced dosages. These are fine.

In addition to having a diet full of antioxidant Superfoods, take the following supplements at a meal early in the day to prime your body in its fight against inflammation. Where two supplements are recommended per day, it is best to take the second one at a later meal to be better absorbed.

Vitamin C (1000 mg/take once a day)—Take vitamin C in the ascorbate form for better absorption. Humans are one of the very few mammals that do not make this vitamin, so it must be obtained through diet and supplements. Vitamin C is essential for cartilage and collagen production, and it is necessary to help vitamin E quench free radicals. Low levels have been associated with inflammatory conditions.

Vitamin E (400 IU/take once a day)—Take vitamin E in the natural "d-alpha, gamma, beta, and delta" mixed forms or as a mix of natural tocopherols and tocotrienols. Vitamin E acts directly as an anti-inflammatory by switching off genes that cause inflammation. It has been found to lower CRP (a blood marker for inflammation) dramatically by blocking free radicals that cause oxidation in the arteries, leading to plaque buildup. Vitamin E has also been found to cut pain levels almost in half in a study of rheumatoid arthritis patients. Since vitamin E has blood-thinning capability, obtain a physician's approval before taking to be sure it will not interfere with medications or medical procedures.

Selenium (100 mg/take once a day)—Selenium is an essential trace mineral deficient in diets around the world where soils are poor in this mineral. It is synergistic with vitamin E, and it is necessary to help the body produce glutathione peroxidase, an important strong antioxidant that the body uses to keep free radicals under control. Selenium may be found in a balanced supplement combination along with vitamin E.

Zinc (10-30 mg/take once a day)—Zinc is required for hundreds of enzymes, especially the enzyme superoxide dismutase, one of the body's natural antioxidants, and for enzymes that make RNA and DNA. Along with vitamin C, zinc has been found to help asthmatics. This mineral may also help to enhance the immune function against colds and flu.

B Complex (50 mg/take twice a day)—The B vitamins perform many important functions in the body. They help to fight stress, support normal immune function, and provide energy. Patients with multiple sclerosis have been found to be usually deficient in B12. Along with folic acid (a B vitamin) and vitamin B6, vitamin B12 is essential for healthy nerve function.

Vitamin D3 (400 IU/take once a day)—As discussed in chapter 6 on vitamin D3, recent scientific studies provide further evidence that it may help to prevent inflammation leading to heart disease. Vitamin D has been found to reduce the autoimmune response in multiple sclerosis patients. We may need to supplement vitamin D levels in our diets, especially in the winter, when those of us living at higher altitudes receive little sunlight on our skin to make vitamin D. New recommendations for daily allowances have been increased to 600 IU for ages one to seventy and to 800 IU for those seventy-one years old and up.

Calcium (1000 mg/take once a day)—Take in a combination supplement also containing magnesium. Calcium is essential for healthy bones, teeth, cardiovascular health, and for restful sleep. Adequate vitamin D is required for absorption of calcium.

Magnesium (500 mg/take once a day)—Magnesium is needed to balance calcium and for cardiovascular and bone health. Deficiencies have been linked to chronic fatigue syndrome, depression, and sleep disturbances. It is best to take magnesium in a balanced supplement also containing calcium.

Fish Oil (1000 mg/take twice a day)—Fish oil capsules contain high concentrations of the omega-3 fatty acids EPA and DHA. As discussed here in chapter 10, omega-3 fatty acids are necessary to maintain an anti-inflammatory diet. Look for supplements with the highest levels of EPA and DHA omega-3 fatty acids.

Alpha-lipoic Acid (100 mg/take once a day)—ALA is both fat and water soluble; therefore, it can act as an antioxidant in every part of the body. It is made in the body, but it may become depleted in times of oxidative stress. It is used in relieving oxidative stress in diabetics, slowing the progression of neuropathy at higher daily dosages (300-600 mg). ALA helps to protect vitamins C and E, making the endogenous antioxidant system more efficient. ALA is important in energy production and possibly helpful in counteracting fatigue.

CHAPTER 12

Practice Breath Work to Reduce Stress and Inflammation

Abundant Evidence

THE MINDFULNESS-BASED STRESS Reduction program begun by Jon Kabat-Zinn in 1979 at the University of Massachusetts Medical Center paved the way for scientific studies on the health benefits of meditative practices involving the breath. Workshops continue to be presented around the country to help patients deal with pain, stress, and many chronic conditions. Early studies of the MBSR program showed that it improved sleep and reduced stress in cancer patients, that meditative-type practices such as yoga and tai chi relieved anxiety and depression and improved sleep in organ transplant patients. The program also improved conditions associated with diabetes, heart disease, and hypertension to name just a few. Benefits were documented, not just by how patients felt, but also by measuring biomarkers, such as blood levels of CRP, a marker for stress and which is associated with systemic inflammation. The common aspect in all meditative-type practices is a mindful focus on controlled breathing.

As previously mentioned, before beginning any of these Breath Work exercises, the GBS patient should obtain medical approval from his or her physician.

Regular Practice Brings Benefits

Although these breathing exercises are not strenuous and they are suitable for any age, it is important to practice according to your comfort level, proceeding only as far as you are ready to go. Establish a Breath Work routine with regular times set aside since consistency is important in generating longer-term benefits. An ultimate goal of a morning and a late-afternoon practice is ideal. Once familiar with the exercises, you can easily do them within a thirty-minute time frame, including the following "Getting Situated."

Getting Situated

The setting is just as important as regular scheduling. In order to meditate on your breath, a quiet area with no distractions should be set aside for your place of practice. Phones should be turned off, and it may be helpful to wear earplugs. You should be seated comfortably, on a chair, on a cushion, on the floor in a cross-legged position, or even on a bed, if necessary, but with your spine erect as if you were suspended from the sky by an invisible string. Then close your eyes and imagine yourself floating on a cloud, releasing all tension in your body. Bring your focus to your breath.

Breath Work Exercises

Each exercise prepares you for the one that follows, so it is important to do them in order.

Exercise 1: *Getting Focused*

This exercise makes use of focused concentration by meditating on your breath. In this exercise, if your mind starts to wander, just gently call attention to your breath, bringing balance to an overactive mind. In the beginning, it is normal for the thoughts of the day to enter and distract you. As you continue to practice, you will find that focusing on the breath will become natural.

Practice these steps for 2-3 minutes:

- Get in a comfortable position and close your eyes or focus on a short distance in front of you.
- Focus on your relaxed breath as it comes and goes.
- Keep your mind on your breath, noticing the flow as it comes and goes.

Exercise 2: *Calming Down*

This exercise begins to reduce stress and anxiety to prepare you for the following exercise. Remember this simple exercise to calm yourself whenever you are in a tense or emotional situation.

Practice these steps for 2-3 minutes:

- Make your breaths deeper by inhaling and exhaling longer.
- Slow down your breaths in and out.
- Now make your breaths more regular and rhythmic.

Exercise 3: *Getting Relaxed*

This exercise is typical of the breathing exercises of Zen meditation. It is very effective in promoting a relaxed state. If you are tired at this point, stop and return to exercise 1 on the next day. You will gradually build up your strength with consistent daily practice.

- Sit or lie in a comfortable position. Place the tip of your tongue on the ridge of the roof of your mouth.
- With your mouth slightly opened and relaxed, comfortably exhale slowly and completely while allowing the exhaled air to make a sound as it is leaving your throat. If you are relaxed properly, the sound should be coming from deep in your throat.
- Gently close your mouth and inhale deep into your belly to the count of four.
- Hold your breath to the count of seven.
- Slowly and evenly exhale to the count of eight.

Repeat these steps two times if you are able. If not, proceed with exercise 4 with the goal of practicing exercise 3 a total of three times.

Exercise 4: *Going Away*

This exercise makes use of what is called guided imagery in meditation. When it is practiced along with Breath Work, it has been shown to be very powerful in promoting relaxation.

- You may change to a more comfortable position. Now imagine that you are lying on a towel on a tropical beach. (The sun is bright, the sand is warm, palm trees are gently blowing in the salty ocean breeze, sea gulls are floating overhead, etc.)

NANCY MOUNT

- Imagine your lungs slowly being inflated by the warm breeze gently blowing off the ocean.
- Imagine that as the waves recede, the air is naturally drawn from your lungs.
- Continue to let the ocean breeze breathe for you as you listen to the waves wash in and out. In with each wave that washes ashore, out with each foamy wave floating out to sea.

Notice how relaxed you feel after these four simple Breath Work practices. Remember that scientific evidence shows that you are not only making a difference in how you feel. You are improving your stress biomarkers and lowering your levels of inflammation, well worth making it part of your daily routine.

AFTERWORD

SCIENTISTS ARE MAKING great strides in identifying the chain of events in the autoimmune reaction of GBS and other polyneuropathies, honing in on the cascade of events that take place during the inflammatory response that causes damage to healthy nerves. Studies worldwide are identifying initiators of the response, locations of the attack, and how free radicals play an integral role in propagating nerve damage. Researchers are making tremendous progress in explaining why the body's immune system mistakes its own healthy cells and tissues as foreign invaders. They are just beginning to understand how the myelin sheath and the nerve axons are repaired once inflammation has subsided. It is the goal of these researchers to share and refine this body of information to develop effective ways for medical intervention to stop GBS in its early stages before extensive nerve damage occurs.

The initial course of development is acute typically, progressing over a course of up to two weeks. This is the crucial stage to make diagnosis to allow medical treatment to begin. Through systematic elimination of other afflictions and reflex testing in combination with nerve conduction tests, treatment can be done if necessary. All of this happens so quickly with great impact on the GBS family and patient. The recovery phase following diagnosis and treatment can be especially difficult because it is essentially a time of waiting to see how quickly and how completely the body heals.

Recognizing that the recovery phase of GBS can be one of great stress and frustration has been my inspiration for writing this book. Through my research on GBS and with my knowledge of the role of antioxidants in inflammation, I became aware that there are actions that can be taken by the patient that are likely to promote recovery. This book is a source that GBS patients and their families can use in learning why antioxidants are key to controlling inflammation and that through something as simple as eating the right foods and adding supplements, recovery may be optimized. That is not to say that a dietary change to predominantly Superfoods may be simple, especially if you have been eating poorly, but consider that perhaps the pro-inflammatory diet predisposed you to acquiring GBS in the first place. Scientific evidence supports a connection between a pro-inflammatory diet and many chronic diseases. After having read this book, you will realize how significant your diet is in controlling inflammation and that the chemicals in healthy foods are nature's medicine.

You have the opportunity to potentially make a real difference in your recovery. When you discover the benefits of regularly eating an abundance of Superfoods and the calming, anti-inflammatory effects of Breath Work, it is my hope that these practices will become your way of life, one that is full of vitality and longevity.

Superfood Recipes to Fit Your Moods

IN CHAPTER 10 a list of "Superfoods" is given to help you in your new meal planning and shopping. These foods high are especially high in antioxidants and nutrients and they are the foods with the greatest ability to help you quench inflammatory free radicals, according to the latest research information. There are certainly others which you may have heard of, such as the exotic acai berries. I do not make the claim that this list is comprehensive, but it is, I believe, a summary of the some of the most highly regarded healthy foods readily available.

The recipes in this Appendix have been organized into four types of appetites, according to how you might be feeling on any particular day, not organized into meal types as breakfast, lunch or dinner. Why should it matter if we prefer to have eggs and whole grain toast for dinner? As long as the daily meals are balanced overall and that you are consistently getting a variety of an abundance of "Superfoods", you will be on your way to helping redirect your immune system.

The following recipes may be altered by substituting one "Superfood" for another or by exchanging herbs and spices. These recipes will not be as effective, however, if important ingredients as found in the list in Chapter 10 are just eliminated. Please use these recipes to guide you in creating your own "Superfood" recipes. Experimenting with new foods, herbs and spices can be a pleasing and satisfying experience. Visualizing the antioxidants at work in your body after a meal can also be very rewarding.

There are six recipes for each of the following mood categories:
- Refreshing and Cooling
- Warm and Comforting
- Flavorful and Savory
- Energizing and Rejuvenating

REFRESHING & COOLING #1

Cold Cumber Soup with Avocado

(4 servings)
2 medium cucumbers, peeled, seeded and cubed
1 cup chicken broth
1 cup plain low fat yogurt
½ avocado, peeled and cubed
2 Tbsp lemon juice
2 Tbsp green onion tops, minced

Blend cubed cucumber just till smooth, being careful to not over blend. Add to a large mixing bowl and stir in broth and yogurt by hand until blended. In a small bowl, sprinkle avocado with lemon juice and toss to coat. Add avocado to cucumber mixture and gently stir. Serve in bowls with green onion garnish on top.

REFRESHING & COOLING #2

Healthy Waldorf Salad

(2 servings)
1 cup chopped celery
1 cup chopped apple
½ cup halved red seedless grapes
1 carrot, peeled and grated
¼ cup canola mayonnaise
1 tsp lemon juice
½ tsp cinnamon
½ cup chopped walnuts
4 cups broken romaine lettuce

In a medium mixing bowl, toss celery, apple, grapes and carrot. Add mayonnaise, lemon juice and cinnamon and toss. Serve on lettuce and sprinkle with walnuts.

*Serve with whole grain bread and extra virgin olive oil for dipping.

REFRESHING & COOLING #3

Turkey Pesto Rolls

(Serves 4)
4 turkey breast cutlets,(approx. ¼" thick)
2 Tbsp canola oil
2 Tbsp canola mayonnaise
2 Tbsp prepared basil pesto
4 large Portobello mushroom slices
2 cups tender greens, e.g., baby lettuce, baby spinach or watercress
4 whole grain sandwich rolls, split and toasted

Heat a medium skillet to medium heat and add canola oil. Pat dry turkey with paper towels and cook 3 minutes. Turn and repeat until turkey is no longer pink in the center. Remove turkey from pan and lightly brown both sides of mushrooms in skillet. Spread mayonnaise on one side of roll and pesto on the other side. Add a layer of greens on the bottom of the roll, then the turkey, a mushroom slice and another layer of greens.

*Serve with cantaloupe slices or another brightly colored fruit.

REFRESHING & COOLING #4

Tuna Rice Salad

(Serves 4)
1 cup brown rice
2 ½ cups chicken broth (without MSG)
2 (6—oz) cans tuna, drained
½ cup minced celery
2 green onions, chopped
2 Tbsp chopped fresh parsley
½ cup dried cranberries
2 Tbsp lemon juice
4 Tbsp olive oil

Add rice to broth and gently simmer for 50 minutes or until liquid is absorbed. Remove from heat and allow to cool. Add remaining ingredients and chill for several hours or overnight.

REFRESHING & COOLING #5

Tropical Fruit Salad with Yogurt

(Makes up to 8 servings)
2 kiwifruit
2 mangoes
1 small papaya, seeded, peeled and cubed
1 cup Greek-style yogurt
1 orange, juiced, seeds removed
1 Tbsp minced mint

Prepare fruit and place in a large bowl. In a small bowl, mix orange juice and yogurt. Serve fruit in bowls with orange yogurt dressing. Sprinkle with mint. (These fruit need time to ripen, so plan ahead.)

REFRESHING & COOLING #6

Herbed Chickpea Sauce on Couscous

(Serves 4)
1 cup chicken broth (MSG-free)
¼ tsp ground allspice
¾ cup whole wheat couscous
1 (19-oz) can chickpeas, rinsed and drained, divided
1/3 cup extra virgin olive oil
¼ tsp cinnamon
¾ tsp dried oregano
2 tsp fresh lemon juice
½ cup finely chopped red onion
½ cup chopped fresh cilantro
½ cup chopped fresh parsley

Combine broth and allspice in saucepan and bring to boil. Stir in couscous, cover and remove from heat. Allow to stand 5 minutes and fluff with fork. To prepare sauce, add half of the chickpeas to a blender and puree slightly. Add the olive oil, the cinnamon and lemon juice and puree until almost smooth. Transfer to a microwaveable medium bowl and stir in the remaining chickpeas, onion, cilantro and parsley. Warm in microwave for 30 seconds and serve on couscous.

WARMING & COMFORTING #1

Walnut Bran Muffins

(Makes 12 regular size muffins)   375 °F, 20 minutes
1 egg, lightly beaten
1 cup skim milk
2 Tbsp canola oil
½ cup wheat bran
1 cup flour (half whole wheat, if desired)
1 Tbsp baking powder
1 tsp cinnamon
¼ cup sugar
½ cup walnuts, broken

Preheat oven to 375 °F. Add egg, milk, oil and bran to a medium mixing bowl and let stand 10 minutes. Add remaining ingredients and stir just to moisten. (Over mixing makes the muffins tough.) Spoon into 12 greased or paper-lined muffin cups and bake approximately 20 minutes.

* Serve with fresh fruit.

WARM & COMFORTING #2

Berry-Oat Crisp

(Serves 4)   400 °F, 30 minutes
2 large baking apples, sliced
2 Tbsp dark brown sugar

1 cup blueberries or blackberries
1 ½ cups rolled oats
1 cup ground almonds (or finely chopped)

Preheat oven to 400 °F. Lightly grease an 8 X 10" baking dish. Place the sliced apple on the bottom of the dish and evenly sprinkle with sugar, then the berries. In a medium bowl, add the oats and almonds and toss. Sprinkle the oil over the oat and almond mix and toss, then spread evenly over the fruit. Bake approximately 30 minutes, until lightly toasted.

WARM & COMFORTING #3

White Bean Soup

3 Tbsp canola oil
1 garlic clove, minced
1 small onion, finely chopped
1 carrot, finely chopped
2 stalks celery, finely chopped
2 cups chopped kale, course stems discarded
8 cups chicken broth
2 (19-oz) cans white beans, drained and rinsed
2 ½ cups whole wheat pasta, cooked and drained
2 Tbsps extra virgin olive oil grated parmesan cheese, to sprinkle

In a large kettle, on medium heat, add canola oil and saute' garlic onion, carrot and celery until onions are translucent, but not browned. Slowly add the chicken broth and bring to a boil. Add the kale and simmer for 10 minutes. Add the cooked pasta and serve in bowls, sprinkled with parmesan cheese, if desired.

* Serve with a crusty bread and extra virgin olive oil sprinkled with dried herbs.

WARMING & COMFORTING #4

Salmon Patties on Buns

(Serves 4)
1 (15-oz) can salmon, undrained
2 large eggs, slightly beaten
½ cup chopped onion
1 cup whole grain bread, cubed
1 Tbsp grated lemon peel
1 Tbsp chopped fresh parsley
4 Tbsp canola oil
½ cup canola mayonnaise
2 Tbsp lemon juice
4 cups romaine lettuce leaves, broken

Empty salmon with juice into large mixing bowl. Using your hands, flake the salmon along with skin (excellent source of additional omega-3 fatty acids), being careful to crush all bones (excellent source of minerals). Form into 8 patties, making them about ½" thick. Heat the oil to medium high in a large fry pan and lightly brown both sides of salmon, about 3 minutes on each side. For the dressing, mix the mayonnaise and lemon juice with a fork until smooth. Serve 2 patties on one cup of lettuce, drizzle with dressing and top with chopped fresh cilantro.

WARM & COMFORTING #5

Egg, Mushroom and Spinach Strata

(Serves 8)   350 °F, 60 minutes
1 (10-oz) package frozen chopped spinach
2 cups whole grain bread cubes
4 large eggs, slightly beaten
2 cups 2% milk
1 cup shredded 2% cheddar cheese

½ tsp prepared mustard
1 Tbsp extra virgin olive oil
1 cup sliced fresh mushrooms

Cook spinach according to directions on the package. Thoroughly drain, squeezing out as much water as possible. Oil a 9" X 13" baking pan and evenly distribute the croutons on the bottom and the spinach on top. In a large bowl, mix the slightly beaten eggs with the milk, mustard and olive oil. Stir in the cheese and pour over the croutons and spinach. Distribute the mushrooms over the top and bake at 350 degrees F for approximately 60 minutes or until a knife inserted in the middle comes out clean.

WARM & COMFORTING #6

Healthy Banana, Walnut & Chocolate Chip Bread

(Makes 1 loaf)   325 °F, 55 minutes
1 ¼ cups all-purpose flour
½ cup whole wheat flour
¼ cup oat bran
1 ½ tsp baking powder
½ tsp baking soda
¼ tsp salt
½ cup sugar
3 large eggs
1/4 cup canola oil
1 tsp vanilla extract
2 large very ripe bananas
½ cup Greek-style yogurt
½ cup chopped dark (at least 50% cacao) chocolate
½ cup chopped walnuts

Oil and flour a 9" X 5" loaf pan. Combine the all-purpose flour, wheat flour, oat bran, baking powder, baking soda and salt. In a large bowl, mix the sugar, eggs, oil and vanilla extract just until blended. Stir in mashed banana and yogurt. Gradually add the dry mixture, stirring just until evenly wet. (Over mixing will make the bread tough.) With a spoon, stir in the chocolate and walnuts. Pour into the prepared pan and bake at 325 °F for approximately 55 minutes, or until a toothpick inserted in the middle comes out clean. Cool in pan for about 20 minutes, then turn out. Delicious warm.

FLAVORFUL & SAVORY #1

Basil Bruchetta

(Serves 6)   350 °F, 10 minutes
6 thick slices crusty bread
¼ cup extra virgin olive oil
6 medium tomatoes, chopped
1 cup fresh sweet basil, torn
4 garlic cloves, minced salt & pepper, to taste

Place the bread slices on a baking sheet. In a medium bowl, combine the remaining ingredients and top the bread slices. Bake at 350 °F for 10 minutes.

FLAVORFUL & SAVORY #2

Pork Chops with Cherries, Apples & Greens

(Serves 4)
3 Tbsp canola oil
4 lean pork chops
1 Tbsp fresh sage, chopped
2 medium apples, unpeeled, sliced ½" thick
4 cups torn cooking greens (e.g., kale, spinach, turnip greens, etc.)
1 orange, juiced, seeded
3 Tbsp grated orange rind

On medium high, heat oil in a heavy skillet or Dutch oven. When hot, add pork and brown on each side then remove to a platter. Lower heat to medium, add other ingredients to the pan juices and braise with a lid on for several minutes until apples are tender, stirring occasionally.

FLAVORFUL & SAVORY #3

Mushroom Rice Bake

(Serves 6) 325 °F, 1 hour
4 Tbsp canola oil
1 medium onion, diced
8 oz fresh mushrooms, sliced
2 ½ cups chicken stock
1 cup uncooked brown rice
2 cloves garlic, minced
½ tsp dried oregano

In a medium saucepan, saute' onions until translucent. Add mushrooms and saute' an additional 2 minutes. Grease a medium size casserole and add stock, rice, garlic and oregano. Stir in the onions and mushrooms. Bake at 325 °F for 1 hour.

FLAVORFUL & SAVORY #4

Sesame Green Beans

(Serves 4)
1 lb fresh green beans, stem ends removed
2 Tbsp sesame oil
1 Tbsp soy sauce (low sodium)
2 Tbsp sesame seeds

Add 4 cups of water to a medium size pot, cover and on medium high heat bring to a rolling boil. Remove the lid and add the beans, bring back to a boil. Cook for only 1 minute. Quickly, drain completely. Toss with oil, soy sauce and sesame seeds.

FLAVORFUL & SAVORY #5

Turkey Breast Cutlets with Herbed Stuffing

(Serves 6)   325 °F, 40 minutes
2 Tbsp canola oil
1 cup chopped onion
½ chopped celery
8 slices whole grain bread, cubed and air-dried overnight
½ tsp poultry seasoning
2 Tbsp chopped fresh parsley
½ cup chicken broth
4 turkey breast cutlets

In a small skillet, saute' the onion and celery in the oil for 2 minutes. Add the bread to a medium size bowl, along with herb seasoning, parsley, broth and onion and celery. Toss to thoroughly mix. Grease an 8" X 8" square glass baking dish. Place the cutlets on the bottom of the dish and evenly distribute the stuffing on top. Cover with foil and bake for 40 minutes.

FLAVORFUL & SAVORY #6

(Serves 4)
2 cups fresh butternut squash, peeled and cubed,
or 2 (10-oz) package frozen cooked squash
3 cups 2% milk
½ tsp cinnamon
¼ tsp nutmeg
¼ tsp ginger
2 Tbsp extra virgin olive oil salt, to taste
½ cup toasted pumpkin seeds or toasted sliced almonds for topping

In a medium saucepan, add the fresh squash to boiling water and cook until soft, drain and mash, or if using frozen squash, heat on low until thawed. Add the milk, cinnamon, nutmeg, ginger, extra virgin olive oil and salt to taste. Heat slowly until hot, but do not boil. Serve in bowls topped with seeds or nuts.

ENERGIZING & REJUVENATING #1

Gingerbread (Made with fresh ginger root)

(Makes 1-9" square cake)   350 °F, 35 minutes
½ cup omega-3 margarine
½ cup brown sugar
1 large egg, well-beaten
1 cup molasses
2 ½ cups flour
1 ½ tsp baking soda
1 tsp cinnamon
1 heaping Tbsp freshly grated ginger
¾ cup hot water

In a large mixing bowl, cream omega-3 margarine and sugar. Add egg and molasses and mix. In a separate bowl, add flour, baking soda and cinnamon and stir by hand to mix evenly. Add the dry ingredients to the creamed mixture. Add hot water and mix until smooth. Pour into a greased 8" or 9" square pan and bake at 350 °F for approximately 35 minutes until a toothpick inserted in the center comes out clean. Serve warm with apple slices and walnuts on the side.

ENERGIZING & REJUVENATING #2

Turkey & Black Bean Chili

(Serves 6)
3 Tbsp canola oil
1 lb ground turkey
2 (15-oz)cans black beans, drained and rinsed
1 medium onion, chopped
2 stalks celery, chopped
3 cloves garlic, minced

2 (28-oz) cans diced tomatoes, with juice
1 Tbsp chopped cilantro
1 Tbsp chili powder
1 tsp dried basil
1 tsp cumin

Heat oil on medium high in a Dutch oven or a large heavy pot and add the ground turkey, broken into pieces. Lightly brown the turkey while stirring and breaking into small pieces. Add the onion and celery, cooking until onions are translucent and the turkey is thoroughly browned. Drain and rinse the beans. Add along with remaining ingredients, cover and simmer for up to 1 hour.

ENERGIZING & REJUVENATING DRINK

Blueberry Protein Slushie

(Serves 2 – 4)
2 cups frozen blueberries
½ cup blueberry juice
1 scoop of soy protein powder
4 – 6 ice cubes

Add all the ingredients to a blender and puree until ice is fine. Pour into glasses.

ENERGIZING & REJUVENATING #3

Easy Chinese Chicken Salad

(Serves 4)
3 cups ready-made rotisserie chicken shredded
3 green onions, thinly sliced
½ cup celery, thinly sliced
½ cup shredded carrot
1 cup watercress leaves, densely packed
2 Tbsp rice wine vinegar

1 Tbsp low sodium soy sauce
1 Tbsp each sesame oil and peanut oil
1 Tbsp grated ginger

In a large bowl, combine the chicken, green onions, celery, carrot and watercress. In a small bowl, whisk together the rice wine vinegar, soy sauce, sesame oil, peanut oil and grated ginger. Pour over the salad, toss and serve.

ENERGIZING & REJUVENATING #4

Tilapia with Lemon Grass and Cucumber Salad

(Serves 4)
2 Tbsp canola oil
4 tilapia filets
2 stalks lemon grass, cut into thin strips or 2 Tbsp jarred lemon grass
2 medium cucumbers, peeled, seeded and thinly sliced
1 cup plain Greek yogurt
1 Tbsp shredded lemon peel

Heat the oil to medium high in a large fry pan. Add the tilapia and cook for 3 minutes, turn and cook for another 3 minutes until lightly brown on each side. Meanwhile, prepare the cucumbers, add to a medium bowl along with the yogurt and lemon peel and toss. Serve on plates with the tilapia, along with the delicious coconut rice (following recipe).

ENERGIZING & REJUVENATING #5

Coconut Rice

(Serves 4)
1 (14-oz) can light coconut milk
½ tsp sea salt
¾ cup brown rice
½ cup chopped fresh cilantro or parsley

Combine all ingredients in a medium saucepan and bring to a simmer over medium heat. Cover with lid, decrease heat to low and simmer for about 30 minutes, or until liquid is absorbed. Add the fresh cilantro or parsley and toss with a fork.

ENERGIZING & REJUVENATING #6

Almond Cookies with Mint Tea

(Makes approximately 6 dozen cookies)   350 °F, 15 minutes
3 cups almond flour
1 cup sugar
2 eggs
1 cup 10X sugar
2 Tbsp loose green tea or 4 green tea bags
2 Tbsp dark brown sugar or 1 ½ Tbsp honey or agave nectar
½ cup fresh mint leaves
6 cups boiling water
2 strips orange peel, white pulp removed

Line 2 large baking sheets with parchment paper. In a large bowl, combine almond flour, sugar and eggs and mix well. Divide dough in half. On a surface lightly dusted with flour, roll each half into a rope that is about 1 ½ " in diameter. Flatten slightly and cut diagonally into 1 ½" slices. Place each slice on its side 1" apart on the baking sheet and bake approximately 15 minutes until pale brown. Remove and cool until just slightly warm. Add 10X sugar to a small paper bag (or plastic container with lid) along with a few cookies at a time a gently shake to coat. Serve along with refreshing mint tea.

For the tea, place the tea leaves into a pre-warmed teapot along with the sugar, mint and orange peel. Pour in the boiling water and steep for 10 minutes. Pour through a strainer into cups to serve hot or allow the tea to cool and pour into ice filled glasses.

SELECTED REFERENCES

Part I

Parry, G. I. and Steinberg, J. S. 2007. *Guillain-Barré Syndrome: From Diagnosis to Recovery.* Saint Paul, MN: AAN Enterprises.

Mayo Clinic. 2010. "Guillain-Barré Syndrome." http://www.mayoclinic.org/guillain-barre/.

Medline Plus Medical Encyclopedia. 2010. "Guillain-Barré Syndrome." http://www.nlm.nih.gov/medlineplus/ency/article/000684.htm.

Trojaborg, W. 1998. Acute and chronic neuropathies: New aspects of Guillain-Barré syndrome and chronic inflammatory demyelinating neuropathy, an overview and an update. *Electroencephalog Clin Neurophysiol* 107 (5): 303-16.

Plomp, J. J. and Willison, H. J. 2009. Pathophysiological actions of neuropathy-related anti-ganglioside antibodies of the neuromuscular junction. *J Physiol* 587 (Pt 16): 3979-99.

National Institute of Neurological Disorders and Stroke. 2010. NINDS Guillain-Barré Syndrome Information Page. http://www.ninds.nih.gov/disorders/gbs/gbs.htm.

Part II

Bromberg, M. B. 2009. Acute neuropathies. *Front Neurol Neurosci* 26: 1-11.

Mc Daneld, L. M., Fields, J. D., Bourdette, D. N. and Bhardwaj, A. 2010. Immunomodulatory therapies in neurologic critical care. *Neurocrit Care* 12 (1): 132-43.

Yuki, N. 2010. Human gangliosides and human lipo-oligosaccharides in the development of human neuropathies. *Methods Mol Biol* 600: 51-65.

Shahrizaila, N. and Yuki, N. 2011. Guillain-barré syndrome animal model: the first proof of molecular mimicry in human autoimmune disorder. *J Biomed Biotechnol* 2011: 829129.

Barbi, F., Ariatti, A., Funakoshi, K., Meacci, M., Odaka, M. and Galassi, G. 2011 Feb 15. (E pub ahead of print). Parvovirus B19 infection antedating Guillain-Barré syndrome variant with prominent facial diplegia. http://www.ncbi.nlm.nih.gov/pubmed/21327846.

Ghabaee, M., Ghanbarian, D., Brujeui, G. N., Bokaei, S., Siavoshi, F. and Gharibzadeh, S. 2010. Could Helicobacter pylori play an important role in axonal type of Guillain-Barré syndrome pathogenesis? *Clin Neurol Neurosurg* 112 (3): 193-8.

Kountouras, J., Zavos, C., Deretzi, G., Gavalas, E., Polyzos, S., Vardaka, E., Kountouras, C., Giartza-Taxidou, E., Koutlas, E. and Tsiptsios, I. 2011. Helicobacter pylori may play an important role in both axonal type Guillain-Barré syndrome and acute inflammatory demyelinating polyradiculoneuropathy. *Clin Neurol Neurosurg.* 113 (6): 520.

Yabe, S., Higuchi, W., Takano, T., Razvina, O., Iwao, Y., Isabe, H. and Yamamoto, T. 2010. In vitro susceptibility to antimicrobial agents and ultrastructural characteristics related to swimming motility and drug action in Campylobacter jejuni and Campylobacter coli. *J Infect Chemother* 16 (3): 174-85.

Kaida, K. and Kusunoki, S. 2010. Antibodies to gangliosides and ganglioside complexes in Guillain-Barré syndrome and Fisher syndrome: Mini-review. *J Neuroimmunol* 223 (1-2): 5-12.

Souayah, N., Nasar, A., Suri, N. F. and Quereshi, Al. 2009. "Guillain-Barré syndrome after vaccination in United States." Data from the Centers for Disease Control and Prevention/Food Drug Administration Vaccine Adverse Event Reporting System (1990-2005). *J Clin Neuromuscul Dis* 11 (1): 1-6.

Loly, J. P., Rikir, E., Seivert, M., legros, E., Defrance, P., Belaiche, J., Moonen, G. and Delwaide, J. 2009. Guillain-Barré syndrome following hepatitis E. *World Gastroenterol* 15 (13): 1645-7.

Islam, Z., Jacobs, B. C., van Belkum, A., Mohammed, Q. D., Islam, M. B., Herbrink, P., Diorditsa, S., Luby, S. P., Talukder, K. A. and Endtz, H. P. 2010. Axonal variant of Guillain-Barré syndrome associated with Campylobacter infection in Bangladesh. *Neurobiol* 74 (7): 581-87.

Ang, C. W., Diijkstra, J. R., deKlerk, M. A., Endtz, H. P., van Doorn, P. A., Jacobs, B. C., Jeurissen, S. H. and Wagenaar, J. A. 2010. Host factors determine anti-GM1 response following oral challenge of chickens with Guillain-Barré syndrome derived Campylobacter jejuni strain GB11. http://www.ncbi.nlm.nih.gov/pmc/articles/PMC2842441.

Sinha, S., Prasas, K. N., Jain, D., Nyati, K. K., Pradham, S. and Agrawal, S. 2010. Immunoglobulin IgG Fc-receptor polymorphisms and HLA class II molecules in Guillain-Barré syndrome. *Acta Neurol Scand* 122 (1): 21-6.

Jiao, H., Wang, W., WangH., Wu, Y. and Wang, L. 2011 May 22 (Epub ahead of print). Tumor necrosis factor alpha 308 G/A polymorphism and Guillain-Barré syndrome risk. *Mol Biol Rep* http://www.ncbi.nlm.nih.gov/pubmed/21604171.

Hardy, C., Lackey, L., Cannon, J., Price, L. and Sibergeld, E. 2011. Prevalence of potentially neuropathic Campylobacter jejuni strains on commercial broiler chicken products. *Int J Food Microbiol* 145 (2-3): 395-9.

Centers for Disease Control and Prevention (CDC). 2009. Safety of influenza A (H1N1) 2009 monovalent vaccines-United States, October 1—November 24, 2009. *Morb Mortal Wkly Rep* 58 (48): 1351-6.

Haber, P., Sejvar, J. M., Kaeloff, Y. and De Sefano, F. 2009.Vaccines and Guillain-Barré syndrome. *Drug Safety* 32 (4): 309-23.

Kuitwaard, K., Bos-Eyssen, M. E., Blomkwist-Markens, P. H. and van Doorn, P. A. 2009. Recurrences, vaccinations and long-term symptoms in GBS and CIDP. *J Peripher Nerv Sys* 14 (4): 310-5.

Gupta, V. and Kohli, A. 2010. Celiac disease associated with recurrent Guillain-Barré syndrome. *Indian Pediatr.* 47 (9): 797-8.

Azhary, H., Farooq, M. U., Bhanushali, M., Majid, A. and Kassab, M. Y. 2010. Peripheral neuropathy: Differential diagnosis and management. *Am Fam Physician* 81 (7): 887-92.

Baheti, N., Manuel, D., Shinde, P., Radhakrishnan, A. and Nair, M. 2010. Hyperreflexic Guillain-Barré syndrome. *Ann Indian Acad Neurol.* 13 (4): 305-7.

Howell, R. J., Davolos, A. G., Clary, M. S., Frake, P. C., Joshi, A. S. and Chaboki, H. 2010. Miller Fisher syndrome presents as an acute voice change to hypernasal speech. *Laryngoscope* 120 (5): 978-80.

Yamazaki, Y., Sugiura, T. and Kurokawa, K. 2010. Abnormal median normal sural sensory response in a patient with an oropharyngeal variant of Guillain-Barré syndrome. *Internal Medicine* 49 (5): 519-20.

George, A. A., Abdurehiman, P. and James, J. 2009. "Finger-drop sign" in Guillain-Barré syndrome. *Neurol India* 57 (3): 282-6.

Scherer, K. 2009. Radial nerve palsy in Guillain-Barré syndrome. *J Clin Neuromuscul Dis* 11 (1): 31-4.

Sejvar, J. J., Lindblade, K. A., Arvelo, W., Padilla, N., Pringle K., Zielinski-Guiterrez, E., Farnon, E., Schonberger, L. B. and Dueger, E. 2010. Clinical assessment of self-representing acute flaccid paralysis in a population-based setting in Guatemala. *Am J Trop Med Hyg* 82 (4): 712-6.

Donofrio, P. D., Berger, A., Brannagan, T. H., Bromberg, M. B., Howard, J. F., Latov, N., Quick, A. and Tandan, R. 2009. Consensus statement: The use of intravenous immunoglobulin in the treatment of neuromuscular conditions report of the AANEM ad hoc committee. *Muscle Nerve* 40 (5): 890-900.

Kuitwaard, K., de Gelder, J., Tio-Gillen, A. P., Hop, W. C., van Gelder, T., van Toorenenbergen, A. W., van Doorn, P. A. and Jacobs, B. C. 2009. Pharmacokinetics of intravenous immunoglobulin and outcome in Guillain-Barré syndrome. *Ann Neurol* 66 (5): 597-603.

Winer, J. B. 2009. When the Guillain-Barré patient fails to respond to treatment. *Pract Neur* 9 (4): 227-30.

Vucic, S., Kiernan, M. C. and Cornblath, D. R. 2009. Guillain-Barré syndrome: an update. *J Clin Neurosci* 16 (6): 733-41.

Hughes, R. A., Swan, A. V., van Doorn, P. A. 2010. Corticosteroids for Guillain-Barré syndrome. Cochrane Database System Rev(2):CD001446.

Usuki, S., Taguchi, K., Thompson, S. A., Chapman, P. B. and Yu, R. K. 2010. Novel anti-idiotype antibody therapy for lipooligosaccharide-induced experimental autoimmune neuritis: Use relevant to Guillain-Barré syndrome. *J Neurosci Res* 88 (8): 1651-63.

Gupta, A., Taly, A. B., Srivastava, A. and Murali, T. 2010. Guillain-Barré syndrome-rehabilitation outcome, residual deficits and requirements for lower limb orthosis at one year follow-up. *Disabil Rehabil* 32 (23): 1897-902.

Bernson, R. A., de Jager, A. E., Kuijer, W., van der Meche," F. G. and Suurmeijer, T. P. 2010. Physchosocial dysfunction in the first year after Guillain-Barré syndrome. *Muscle Nerve* 41 (4): 533-9.

De Vries, J. M., Hagemans, M. L., Bussmann, J. B., van der Ploeg and van Doorn, P. A. 2010. Fatigue in neuromuscular disorders: Focus on Guillain-Barré syndrome and Pompe diseases. *Cell Mol Life Sci* 67 (5): 701-13.

Elgert, G. and Olmstead, L. 1999. The treatment of chronic inflammatory demyelinating polyradiculoneuropathy with acupuncture: A clinical case study. *Am J Acupunct* 27 (1-2): 15-21.

Nakano, T., Chang, Y. F., Lai, C. Y., Hsu, L. W., Chang, Y. C., Deng, J. Y., Huang, Y. Z., Honda, H., Chen, K. D. and Wang, C. C. 2010 Dec 21. (E pub ahead of print). Impact of artificial sunlight therapy on the progress of non-alcoholic fatty liver disease in rats. *J Hepatol* http://www.ncbi.nlm.nih.gov/pubmed/21184788.

Chen, A. C., Huang, Y. Y., Sharma, S. K. and Hamblin, M. R. 2011 Jan 8. (E pub ahead of print). Effects of 810-nm laser on murine bone-marrow derived dendritic cells. *Photomed Laser Surg* http://www.ncbi.nlm.nih.gov/pubmed/21214383.

Matthews, K. A., Zheng, H., Kravitz, H. m., Sowers, M., Bromberger, J. T., Buyesse, D. J., Owens, J. F., Sanders, M. and Hall, M. 2010. Are inflammatory and coagulation biomarkers related to sleep characteristics in mid-life women? Study of Women's Health Across the Nation Sleep Study. *Sleep* 33 (12): 1649-55.

Nyati, K. K., Prasad, K. N., Verma, A. and Paliwab, V. K. 2010. Correlation of matrix metaloproteinases-2 and—9 with pro-inflammatory cytokines in Guillain-Barré syndrome. *J Neurosci Res* 88 (16): 3540-6.

Zhang, H. L., Wu, J. and Zhu, J. 2010. The role of apolipoprotein E in Guillain Barré syndrome and experimental autoimmune neuritis. *J Biomed Biotechnol* 2010: 357412.

Xia, R. H., Yosel, N. and Ubogu, E. E. 2010. Selective expression and cellular localization of pro-inflammatory chemokine ligand/receptor pairs in the sciatic nerve of a severe murine experimental autoimmune neuritis model of Guillain Barré syndrome. *Neuropathol Appl Neurobiol* 36 (57): 388-98.

Molendi-Coste, O., Legry, V. and Leclercq, I. A. 2011. Why and how meet n-3 PUFA dietary recommendations? *Gastroenterol Res Pract* 2011: 364040.

Halade, G. V., Williams, P. J., Lindsey, M. L. and Fernandes, G. 2011. Fish oil decreases inflammation and reduces cardiac remodeling in rosiglitazone treated aging mice. *Pharmacol Res* 63 (4): 300-7.

Schwartz, J., Dube, K., Alexy, U., Kalhoff, H. and Kersting, M. 2010. PUFA and LC-PUFA intake during the first year of life: Can dietary practices achieve a guideline diet? *Eur J Clin Nutr* 64 (2): 124-30.

Bousserouel, S., Broillet, A., Raymondjean, M. and Andreani, M. 2003. Different effects of n-6 and n-3 polyunsaturated fatty acids on the activation of rat smooth muscle cells by interleukin-1 beta. *J Lipid Res* 44 (3): 601-11.

San Giovanni, J. P. and Chew, E. Y. 2005. The role of omega-3 long-chain polyunsaturated fatty acids in health and disease of the retina. *Prog Retin Eye Res* 24 (1): 87-138.

Talhouk, R. S., Karam, C., Fostok, S., El Jouni, W. and Barbour, E. K. 2007. Anti-inflammatory bioactivities in plant extracts. *J Med Food* 10 (1): 1-10.

Clutterbuck, A. L., Mobasheri, A., Shakibaei, M., Allaway, D. and Harris, P. 2009. Interleukin-1 beta-induced extracellular matrix degradation and glycosaminoglycan release is inhibited by curcumin in an explant model of cartilage inflammation. *Ann N Y Acad Sci* 1171: 428-35.

Xia, X., Ling, W., Ma, J., Xia, M., Hou, M., Wang, Q., Zhu, H. and Tang, Z. 2006. An anthocyanin-rich extract from black rice enhances atherosclerotic plaque stabilization in apolipoprotein—E—deficient mice. *JNutr* 136 (8): 2220-5.

Mauray, A., Felgines, C., Morand, C., Mazur, A., Scalbert, A. and Milenkovic, D. 2010. Nutrigenomic analysis of the protective effects of bilberry anthocyanin-rich extract in apo-E deficient mice. *Genes Nutr* 5 (4): 343-53.

Chung, E. Y., Kim, B. H., Hong, J. T., Lee, C. K., Ahn, B., Nam, S. Y., Han, S. B. and Kim, Y. 2010 Dec 27 (E pub ahead of print). Resveratrol down-regulates interferon-gamma-inducible inflammatory genes in macrophages: Molecular mechanism via decreased STAT-1 activation. *J Nut Biochem* http://www.ncbi.nlm.nih.gov/pubmed/21189227.

Aziz-Seible, R. S., Lee, S. M., Kharbauda, K. K., McVicker, B. L. and Casey, C. A. 2011. Ethanol feeding potentiates the pro-inflammatory response of Kupffer cells to cellular fibronectin. *Alcohol Clin Exp Res* 35 (4): 717-25.

Jablonski, J. L., Chonchol, M., Pierce, G. L., Walker, A. Z. and Seals, D. R. 2011. 25-Hydroxyvitamin D deficiency is associated with inflammation-linked vascular endothelial dysfunction in middle-aged and older adults. *Hypertension* 57 (1): 63-9.

Adorini, L. and Penna, G. 2009. Induction of tolerogenic dendritic cells by vitamin D receptor agonists. *Handb Exp Pharmacol* (188): 251-73.

Takeda, M., Yamashita, T., Sasaki, N., Nakajima, K., Kita, T., Shinohara, M., Ishida, T. and Hirata, K. 2010. Oral administration of an active form of vitamin D3 (calcitrol) decreases atherosclerosis in mice by inducing regulatory T cells and immature dendritic cells with tolerogenic functions. *Atheroscler Thromb Vas Biol* 30 (12): 2495-503.

Chen, Y., Kong, J., Sun, T., Li, G., Szeto, F. L., Liu, W., Deb, D. K., Wang, Y., Zhao, Q and Thadhani, R. 2010. 1, 25-dihydroxyvitamin D3 suppresses inflammation-induced expression of plasminogen activator inhibitor-1 by blocking nuclear factor-kappa beta activation. *Arch Biochem Biophys* 507 (2): 241-7.

Strohle, A., Wolters, M. and Hahn, A. 2010. Micronutrients at the interface between inflammation and infection ascorbic acid and calciferol: Part 2: Calciferol and the significance of nutrient supplements. *Inflamm Allergy Drug Targets* 10 (1): 64-74.

Khoo, A. L., Chai, L. Y., Koenen, H. J., Kullberg, B. J., Joosten, I., van der Ven, A. J. and Netea, M. G. 2011. 1, 25-Dihydroxyvitamin D3 modulates cytokine production induced by Candida *albicans*: Impact of seasonal variations of immune responses. *J Infect Dis* 203 (1): 122-30.

Ghibu, S., Richard, C., Vergely, C., Zeller, M., Cottlin, Y. and Rochette, L. 2009. Antioxidant properties of an endogenous thiol: Alpha-lipoic acid, useful in the prevention of cardiovascular diseases. *J Cardiovasc Pharmacol* 54 (5): 391-8.

Shay, K. P., Moreau, R. F., Moreau, R. F., Smith E. J., Smith A. R., Hagen, T. M. 2009. Alpha-lipoic acid as a dietary supplement: Molecular mechanisms and therapeutic potential. *Biochim Biophys Acta* 1790 (10): 1149-60.

Maczurek, A. Hager, K., Kenklies, M., Sharman, M., Martins, R., Engel, J., Carlson, D. A. and Munch., G. 2008. Lipoic acid as an anti-inflammatory and neuroprotective treatment for Alzheimer's disease. *Adv Drug Deliv Rev* 60 (13-14): 1463-70.

Part III

Balch, James F. 1998. *The Superantioxidants: Why They Will Change the Face of Healthcare in the 21st Century.* New York: M. Evans and Company, Inc.

Challam, Jack. 2003. *The Inflammation Syndrome.* Hoboken, New Jersey: Wiley & Sons, Inc.

Packer, Lee and Colman, Carol. 1999. *The Antioxidant Miracle.* New York: John Wiley & Sons, Inc.

Oh, B., Butow, P., Mullan, B., Clarke S., Beale, P., Pavlakis, N., Kothe, E., Lam, L. and Rosenthal, D. 2010. Impact of medical qigong on quality of life, fatigue, mood and inflammation in cancer patients: A randomized controlled trial. *Ann Oncol* 21 (3): 608-14.

Scmidt, S., Grossman, P., Schwarzer, B., Jena, S., Naumann, J. and Walach, H. 2011. Treating fibromyalgia with mindfulness-based stress reduction: results from a 3-armed randomized controlled trial. *Pain.* 152 (2): 361-9.

Pullen, P. R., Nagamia, S. H., Mehta, P. K., Thompson, W. R., Bernadot, D., Hammoud, R., Parrott, J. M., Sola, S. and Khan, B. V. 2008. Effects of yoga on inflammation and exercise capacity in patients with chronic heart failure. *J Card Fail* 14 (5): 407-13.

Kim, K. S., Lee, S. W., Choe, M. A., Yi, M. S., Choi, S. and Kwon, S. H. 2005. Effects of abdominal breathing training using biofeedback on stress, immune response and quality of life in patients with a mastectomy for breast cancer. *Taehan Kanhee Hakhoe Chi* 35 (7): 1295-303.

Olivo, E. L. 2009. Protection throughout lifespan: The psychoneuroimmunologic impact of Indo-Tibetan meditative and yogic practices. *Ann NY Acad Sci* 1172: 163-71.

Greeson, J. M. 2009. Mindfulness research update: 2008. *Complement Health Pract Rev* 14 (1): 10-18.

Creswell, J. D., Hector, F. M., Cole, S. W. and Irwin, M. R. 2009. Mindfulness meditative training effects on CD4+ T lymphocytes in HIV-1 infected adults: A small randomized controlled trial. *Brain Behav Immun* 23 (2): 184-188.

Ozkul, A., Ayhan, M., Yenisey, C., Akyol, A., Guney, E. and Ergin, F. A. 2010. The role of oxidative stress and endothelial injury in diabetic neuropathy and neuropathic pain. *Neuro Endocrinol Lett* 31 (2): 261-4.

Ziegler, D., Sohr, C. G. and Nourooz-Zadeh, J. 2004. Oxidative stress and antioxidant defense in relation to the severity of diabetic polyneuropathy and cardiovascular autonomic neuropathy. *Diabetes Care* 27 (9): 2178-83.

Iqbal, R., Mughal, M. S., Arshad, N. and Arshad, M. 2010. Pathophysiology and antioxidant status of patients with fibromyalgia. *Rheumatol Int* 31 (2): 149-52.)

De La Hoz, C. L., Castro, F. R., Santos, L. M. and Langone, F. 2010. Distribution of inducible nitric oxide synthase and tumor necrosis factor-alpha in the peripheral nervous system of Lewis rats during ascending paresis and spontaneous recovery from experimental autoimmune neuritis. *Neuroimmunomodulation.* 17 (1): 56-66.

Conti, G., Rostami, A., Scarpini, E., Baron, P.,Galimberti, D., Bresolini, N., Contri, M., Palumbo, C. and De Poi, A. 2004. Inducible nitric oxide synthase (i NOS) in immune-mediation demyelination and Wallerian degeneration of the rat peripheral nervous system. *Exp Neurol.* 187 (2): 350-8.

Dogonadze, S. I., Ninua N. G., Gordeziani, M. G., Kavlashvili, M. S. and Sanikidze, T. V. 2006. The role of oxidative stress in the pathogenesis of GBS. *Georgian Med News.* 140: 43-7.

Darley-Usmar, V. and Halliwell, B. 1996. Blood radicals: reactive nitrogen species, reactive oxygen species, transition metal ions and the vascular system. *Pharm Res* 13 (5): 649-62.

Kumar, K. T., Chandrika, A., Sumanth, K. N., Sireesha, P., Rao, S. and Rao, A. 2004. Free radical toxicity and antioxidants in Guillain-Barré syndrome, a preliminary study. *Clin Chim Acta* 346 (2): 205-9.

Surapaneni, K. M. and Venkataramana, G. 2007. Status of lipid peroxidation, glutathione, ascorbic acid, vitamin E and antioxidant enzymes in patients with osteoarthritis. *Indian J Med Sci* 61 (1): 9-14.

Redford, E. J., Kapoor, R. and Smith, K. J. 1997. Nitric oxide donors reversibly block axonal conduction: demyelinated axons are especially susceptible. *Brain* 120 (Pt 12): 2149-57.

Shrager, P., Custer, A. W., Kazarinova, K., Rasband, M. N. and Mattson, D. 1998. Nerve conduction block by nitric oxide that is mediated by the axonal environment. *J Neurophysiol* 79 (2): 529-36.

Gutowski, N. J., Pinkham, J. M., Akanmu, D., Chirico, S. and Murphy, R. P. 1998. Free radicals in inflammatory neurological disease: increased lipid peroxidation and haptoglobulin levels in Guillain-Barré syndrome. *Ir J Med Sci* 167 (1): 43-6.

Hartung, H. P., Jung, S., Stoll, G., Zielasek, J., Schmidt, B., Archelos, J. J. and Toyka, K. V. 1992 Inflammatory mediators in demyelinating disorders of the CNS and PNS. *J Neuroimmunol* 40 (2-3): 197-210.

Smith, K. J., Kapoor, R., and Felts, P. A. 1999. Demyelination: the role of reactive oxygen and nitrogen species. *Brain Pathol* 9 (1): 69-92.

Part IV

Challem, Jack. 2003. *The Inflammation Syndrome.* Hoboken, New Jersey: Wiley & Sons, Inc.

Weil, A. 2000. *Eating Well for Optimum Health: The Essential Guide to Food, Diet and Nutrition.* New York: Alfred A. Knopf.

Fjorback, L., Arendt, M., Ombol. E. Fink, P. and Walach, H. 2011 Apr 28. (Epub ahead of print) Mindfulness-based stress reduction and mindfulness-based cognitive therapy—a systematic review of randomized controlled trials. *Acta Psychiatr Scand* http://www/ncbi/nlm/nih.gov/pubmed/21534932.

INDEX

M

magnesium, 57, 59-61
Miller Fisher syndrome (MFS), 16, 18, 87
Mindfulness-Based Stress Reduction (MBSR), 46-47, 62, 92-93
molecular mimicry, 26, 85
myelin sheath, 14, 17-18

N

nerve axon, 14, 18
nerve conduction studies (NCS), 16, 18, 27-28
nonfoods, 54
nonsteroidal anti-inflammatory drugs (NSAIDS), 21
nutraceuticals, 15, 51

O

omega-3, 34-35, 42, 52-53, 61, 90
omega-6, 34-35, 52-53
omega-9, 52
oxidative stress, 43-44, 61, 92

P

paresthesia, 14, 16-17
peripheral nervous system, 13-14
physical therapy, 20, 22
plasmapheresis, 21
polyphenols, 35, 54
positive pressure ventilation (PPV), 20
pranayama, 45
ptosis, 18

Q

qigong, 46, 91

R

resveratrol, 36, 90

S

Selenium, 59-60
stress, definition of, 46
Superfoods, 9, 15, 37-38, 51-52, 59
  beans, 55, 57
  dark chocolate, 58
  drinks, 57
  fish, 57
  fruits, 57
  herbs and spices, 57
  nuts and seeds, 57
  vegetables, 57
  whole grains, 57
Super Mood Food, 38, 58
superoxide dismutase, 60

T

tai chi, 46, 62
type 2 diabetes, 54

V

vitamin C, 59
vitamin D3, 36, 60, 90
vitamin E, 60

Y

yoga, 45-47, 62, 92

Z

zinc, 59-60

www.ingramcontent.com/pod-product-compliance
Lightning Source LLC
Chambersburg PA
CBHW022113170526
45157CB00004B/1613